The Aargh to Zen of Perimenopause

Disclaimer

All views and opinions are those of the chapter authors. The information contained in this book is not intended to replace the advice or recommendations of your primary health care provider, and is not intended as medical advice. Please consult your doctor before starting anything new.

The Aargh to Zen of Perimenopause

The Essential Guide to Navigating Perimenopause Your Way

Emily Barclay and The Perimenopause Hub Experts

Kirsten Alberts

Susannah Alexander

Tina Belt

Julie Blatherwick

Annika Carroll

Toni Chambers

Hannah Charman

Dominique Cocuzza

Sophia Cleverly

Denise Drinkwalter

Eleanor Duelley

Nikki Faldo

Denise Fitzpatrick

Rebecca Franklin

Kathy Fritz

Julie Ann Garrido

Debi Haden

Naomi Harris

Sahar Hooti

Victoria Howell

Geraldine Joaquim

Helen Jones

Jo Jones

Caroline Kerslake

Suzanne Laurie

Andrea Marsh

Dr Tanya McEachern

Michaela Newsom

Nic Pendregaust

Kekezza Reece

Emma Roache

Marcelle Rose

Ruby Saharan

Tracy Seider

Tanya Stricek

Nicola Travlos

Dr Susanna Unsworth

Laura Viale

Polly Warren

Book Cover Design: Jack Stevens
Editing: Emily Barclay
Typesetting / Proofreading: Emily Barclay
Publishing: Emily Barclay

Dedication

This book wouldn't have been possible without the help of our team of experts (they hate being called that) and there's simply not enough space here in print for me to explain how qualified they are to have contributed to this manual... so I won't try.

Scan the QR code to take a much closer look at each member of the team.

The book is also dedicated to all the perimenopausal women who make up our lovely Perimenopause Hub community.

You're all epic, don't ever forget that.

Meet The Experts

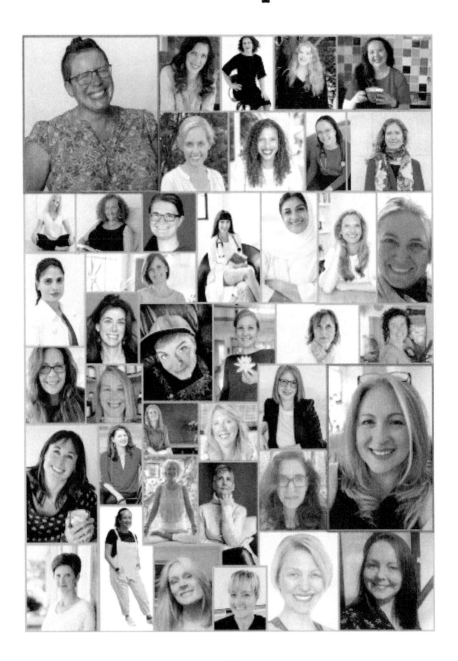

Introduction

Hi, I'm Emily, your peri-godmother. I started experiencing perimenopause symptoms when I was 39. At that time, I was training for Ironman triathlons. I was the fittest I've ever been. Yet all of a sudden I was exhausted, angry, tearful, gaining weight. I didn't recognise who I was becoming, and I desperately tried to fight it.

It took 13 doctor visits before I got the word perimenopause. I came out of that appointment feeling like a weight had lifted because I finally had an explanation for why I was changing, I had something to look up, I could go and find support groups. I found great relief in realising that if I had survived puberty, I would probably manage to get through this reverse puberty.

I came home and looked for the resources I wanted. I found online groups for women in menopause, but they all seemed to have reached the magic point of having finished their periods. They were mostly in their 50s, talking about things that bore little relation to my 42-year old self.

I found websites from individual practitioners claiming they had THE answer to managing my peri/menopause symptoms. I was sceptical, to be honest – how could there be just one way to navigate this when all of us, by the time we reach our 40s, have a totally different life story, a different medical history, a different outlook on how we want to manage our health.

Since by this point I was no longer Ironman training, I had a bit of spare time and figured I could bring together experts from around the world to help women in the way they want to be helped. And thus the Perimenopause Hub was born. We now have a panel of around 55 experts, from around the world, ranging from doctors to Chinese Medicine specialists to counsellors, nutritionists and more. There is someone for everyone.

This is the Hub in book form. You can dip in to find the help, support, information you need right now. And next month, when you need something else, you can dip in again. And again. And again.

You'll notice each expert has a flag on her headshot photo - this is to let you know which version of English they use (and for the most part which country they are based in).

We, the authors and me, are here for you, in this book, whenever you need us. And if you enjoy someone's advice, you'll find an email address or QR code at the end of their chapter via which you can make contact. Please do reach out if you'd like to work with any of the experts. They are all wonderful at what they do (yes, I'm biased, but it's true).

Go read, learn, enjoy.

Contents

CHAPTER ONE
Your Body is a System: Using Acupuncture, Herbs and Supplements for a Natural Transition through Perimenopause by Tina Belt, L.Ac. Dipl OM, Functional Medicine Practitioner

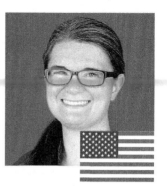

Bio: Tina is a Natural Functional Medicine Practitioner who lives and practices in Lakewood, Colorado in the United States. She and her husband love to hike, and their two boys love to be silly, video game and play soccer. Tina's practice includes patients of all ages and for more information and help you can visit HormonaltoHappy.com to see her online programs for Perimenopause and to find out more information about working with her.

Business: Good Needles
Website: www.goodneedles.com

As a practitioner of Herbal Medicine and an Acupuncturist for the last 14 years, when my own Perimenopause knocked me over, I immediately put together an herb and supplement plan. I explained to my husband my mood swings, lack of libido, painful intercourse, and night sweating. Even being an expert, I experienced the stress and suffering of sleepless nights and the difficulty of having faith in a plan. I do not want you to suffer. You can support and nourish your body, your glands, and create enough hormones to stop having symptoms and transition naturally to Menopause. There is hope and I am going to give you tweaks I use with my patients, a lifestyle plan and the understanding of how your body works in systems in order to heal fully.

Part 1: Understanding Your Body Systems for Deeper, More Complete Healing

The topic I chose is a complex one. Your body works as a system. I tell women to explain to their husband that they are like a car that goes for a service at the garage. You and your husband want to hear that the oil needs changing and that is all. However, that is not all. Your radiator needs flushing, your timing belt is about to snap. Your shocks are worn. Your female body is the most complex system in your household and the most in need of attention at this point.

Men make their hormones from the testicles their whole life. While they have similar andropause issues or low testosterone and they have some of the same steps I am about to go through to correct their problems, essentially it is easier for me to fix my male clients. It takes less time to get them feeling better. They really struggle to understand that the extra task or the hard day at work literally mean you have less estrogen that night! I used to joke with my husband that foreplay is doing the dishes. Foreplay is not asking me to have sex so I can have some sense of control about how I feel and if I have enough hormones and energy to WANT to.

The systems involved in your hormones are:

1.The Brain

We have many estrogen receptors in the brain, meaning as it declines, many women feel depressed, discover they have ADHD, or their brain fog is so bad they feel they are losing their minds or can no longer work. Some experience debilitating headaches. During perimenopause, there must be enough adrenal hormones to make your estrogen, progesterone and testosterone. Your brain is signaling your ovaries to ovulate. Your adrenal and thyroid glands are on the feedback loop too, known as the HPA axis or the HPT Axis, the brain is telling your glands and organs how to function.

When the ovaries are not responding, the volume in the HPA and HPT axis is essentially turned up too high, leading to anxiety, difficulty sleeping, worsening headaches and changes in your cycles.

Brain Fog is often supported by adding Gingko Biloba to your supplement plan.

2.The Digestive System

Because perimenopausal symptoms are so stressful, they often lower stomach acid. I often end up adjusting a stomach that is tight and pulling up. B vitamins keep the stomach valve closed between the epigastrium and the esophagus. Many women experience an over acid stomach with burning at the epigastrium or they experience low or high appetite and inflammation that comes with bloating after a meal.

- Take B vitamins at breakfast and lunch to keep the stomach closed. Only eat whole grains when you are craving them, such as quinoa or brown rice.
- Eliminate crackers or chips.
- Get extra protein. I keep trail mix around and a nut bowl, so that I reach for that instead of sugar.
- Add fermented foods like sauerkraut.

Patient story

I recently had a young teacher with IBS in her 30's who came to see me due to night sweating. Her night sweating resolved with the Mediherb liquid extract of chamomile. This is a pharmaceutical grade herbal extract, so much stronger than a regular cup of tea. However, the point is that I resolved her hormonal issue by improving her digestion.

3. The Liver and Gallbladder

These two organs are extremely important for women to manage their weight in menopause. The bigger belly we see can indicate the formation of gallstones or thick bile. Bile should be a liquid that squirts into the stomach when we eat fats.

I usually start with a cleanse to thin the bile and heal the liver if warranted, but how do you know if it is warranted?
A large belly indicates that you need to cleanse the Liver and Gallbladder!

The liver breaks down excessive hormones. Any ladies struggling with unwanted large breast growth or tingling nipples or excessively tender breasts are in desperate need of a cleanse. I use Standard Process's cleanse products.

When embarking on a cleanse, it is absolutely critical that you continue to have regular bowel movements. If you do not, then stop or add fiber to help get those toxins out.

4.Thyroid

The thyroid is a very, very important piece of that hormonal weight gain puzzle. Many women have high and low thyroid symptoms at the same time, and the detoxification I do helps to get plastics and halogens out of the thyroid ports. Then I gently bring some iodine and selenium in to nourish the organ. Healing the thyroid takes time and will not cause weight loss immediately, but once the thyroid is working right, the weight should just come off.

In my case, I supported my thyroid for several months with iodine and then dropped 13 pounds easily and with no change to exercise.

Part 2: Supplements

I LOVE herbs and supplements. They are my favorite and the older I get the more I lean into them.

1. A B complex is critical and taking more than one a day is helpful. You know you need a B complex if you are weeping all the time, if you have nerve issues, or if you are tired. We do not store b vitamins and the more stressed we are, the more

we burn through them.

2. The second most common thing I put my patients on is **magnesium.** Magnesium helps you with constipation, it helps you with muscle tics, twitches and cramps and it helps you with muscular tension. Stress and sugar deplete magnesium. Each day you may need a different amount. Taking a supplement at bedtime can really help with restless legs or waking up with muscle cramps.

Be mindful that too much magnesium will cause a loose stool
.

* Note of caution – for my patients with potassium deficiency too, then supplementing with magnesium alone can cause heart palpitations. If you develop heart palpitations, then you need to eat more potassium foods, take a potassium supplement, or have an electrolyte drink.

3. An **estrogen herb formula** is critical. I use Mediherb Femco and Mediherb Wild Yam Complex. There are many herbs that help to increase estrogen. If you are already taking black cohosh, ashwagandha or one of the menopause formulas on the shelf, then you have this supplement covered. Be sure to take it regularly and at the recommended dosage for at least 3 months to evaluate if it is helping.

4. The fourth supplement I LOVE is a **zinc, copper and iron** blend called Chezyn from Standard Process. Essentially, if you are still menstruating, then I want to replace the lost blood every month. Having a period takes a lot of energy. The

closer you get to menopause, the more work it is for your body to have a cycle. So be kind to your body.

How to start your supplement plan:
Even if you take a multivitamin, I want you to have a separate magnesium and B complex. Even if you love to take B6 or B12, I want you to have a separate B complex.

Breakfast: Multivitamin, hormonal support supplement, B complex
Lunch: Hormonal supplement and B complex and Chezyn or iron supplement
Dinner or bedtime: Magnesium supplement

If you stick with it, you should feel calmer and sane at about 2 weeks and your symptoms should be easing at about 3 months. If you are replacing your hormones naturally, then you will stay on your hormonal supplement until you are able to come off it without a return of symptoms like hot flashes and night sweating. It is ok to continue on with natural hormonal supplements at a maintenance dose as long as necessary.

It takes 3-6 months to shift your hormones, so be patient. What I put down above is basic. Every time you have a period, you may feel like you have backslid. Every time you are hit with extra stress, you may feel worse. Every time you overwork and have a big day, you may feel worse. And every time you take your supplements you are refueling!

Part 3: Creating More Space to Take Care of YOU

Being a woman in perimenopause can be challenging, because the two key things that will help you a lot are hard to do. One is to minimize stress. The other is to rest more. This is because your hormones are now converting from your adrenal glands and overwork decreases their availability. Stress hijacks them and creates cortisol.

Use the notes section to do this exercise:

1.   Make a list of things that fill you up and make you have more energy.

2.   Make a list of things that you resent or are frustrated with or do not enjoy.

3.   Spend a little time looking at these lists. What do you want to change first to feel better?

In Summary

With my patients, I love to get the body completely functional and set up for long term health.

Consider Acupuncture to help calm your nervous system, stop heavy periods, shrink fibroids, get rid of your hot flashes and more. In school one of my teachers said, "You Americans all have the problem. In China we do not have the problem."

Herbal formulas in Traditional Chinese Medicine can stop those cramps or slow that heavy bleeding or ease your anxiety and they work to help the body heal and not just mask your symptoms.

The basics I discussed above will serve you well if you implement them and reduce or eliminate many of your symptoms over time. At any point that you feel overwhelmed, seeking out a trained professional will help you to accomplish your goal of feeling your best and transitioning to menopause naturally. You may also need to seek out help if you have diabetes, high blood pressure, hyperthyroidism or autoimmune diseases. The protocols suggested are deemed safe and appropriate for most people.

It is not uncommon for me to have patients drag all their supplements in and evaluate them for overdoses of certain vitamins. Even though we do not store our B vitamins, too much B vitamin at ONE time can create high blood pressure, especially if they are combined with mushrooms, for example, which are already high in b vitamins.

Scan the QR code to find out how you can go from hormonal to happy.

Notes/Journalling Page

1.   Make a list of things that fill you up and make you have more energy.

2.   Make a list of things that you resent or are frustrated with or do not enjoy.

3.   Spend a little time looking at these lists. What do you want to change first to feel better?

CHAPTER TWO
Perimenopause & Alcohol
don't make a good cocktail
by Dominique Cocuzza

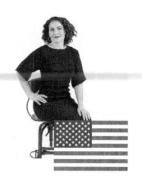

Bio: Dominique Cocuzza is a 51-year-old perimenopausal woman devoted to helping women Age Better and reduce Peri/Menopause symptoms through lifestyle interventions. She is the CEO of a tech start-up called NuAge that is building a menopause app. As a Certified Menopause Coaching Specialist, she has improved the lives of over 1,000 women by helping them build better habits with food, fitness, lifestyle, and mindset. Dominique resides in Charlottesville, Virginia, and can be reached at dominique@nu-age.net

Business: NuAge
Website: www.nu-age.net

Drinking while perimenopausing is dangerous

As you embark on the sometimes rough sea of change that is perimenopause, I invite you to join me on a personal exploration of a topic that has shaped my own journey: alcohol. Here we will navigate the intricate waters of hormones, liver health, well-being, and the profound impact our choices have on our long-term health outcomes.

The Sign of the Times

Picture this – a beautiful evening spent with a close friend at a charming vineyard. Laughter, stories, and a bottle of wine shared in the glow of friendship. Then... the day after... As I opened my eyes the next morning, I felt like I had been hit by a truck and was bedridden all day. This unwelcome day of rest was actually one of the 1st signals that my body was undergoing changes beneath the surface.

I was 46 years old and I found myself in a sudden crisis of confidence along with other disturbing changes. I began to wonder if I was losing my mind. My PMS was at an all-time high, and I was an irritated and anxious mess. My breasts were very tender and seemed to grow by the day. I knew something was wrong when I found myself getting lost while driving to familiar places.

I was terrified. I thought I was going into Alzheimer's. Over the course of 2 years, I visited my gynecologist looking for answers. Was this perimenopause? "You are not there yet," she kept telling me since I was having regular periods and no hot flashes.

High WHAT?

My doctor finally agreed to hormonal testing on visit 4 when

I showed up at her office hysterically crying. Both she and I were confused when we discovered that my estrogen level was over 1500 pg/ml (normal range is <50). No… I was not pregnant. It was perimenopause.

"How could this be?" I thought. I was one of those biohacking geeks who began optimizing for my menopause at 40. I thought I was going to glide into menopause. I read the books, made lifestyle changes, and was doing "all the things." I expected my levels of estrogen to be lower than normal.

Too much of a good thing

So I went back to the books to study high estrogen in perimenopause, particularly the pioneering work of Dr. Jerilynn Prior[1]. Here's the short story. Estrogen and progesterone are the primary female sex hormones produced in the ovaries. During our fertile years, our ovaries produce progesterone when we ovulate. As we go through perimenopause, we experience irregularities in our ovulation. Sometimes more eggs are "recruited" each cycle, causing estrogen levels to rise higher than normal[2]. At other times we don't ovulate and we don't produce progesterone as a result. Unpredictable cycles in perimenopause leave us with too much estrogen relative to progesterone.

This is called "estrogen dominance", which is quite common in perimenopause. Women experience 20-30% higher levels of estrogen in perimenopause, and our estrogen levels

1. The Centre for Menstrual Cycle and Ovulation Research: https://www.cemcor.ca/about-us
2. Science Direct - Women's Reproductive System: https://www.sciencedirect.com/science/article/pii/S174067572030013X

fluctuate much more widely[3]. More estrogen might sound like a good thing since we hear so much about "estrogen deficiency" leading up to menopause, but estrogen dominance can give rise to a myriad of symptoms – from weight gain to heavy or frequent periods, from enlarged to painful and fibrocystic breasts. Other signs of high estrogen include mood swings, headaches, low sex drive, and forgetfulness. Yup, I had all of these.

Wake Up Call

That single blood test changed the course of my life. I began a systematic audit of my lifestyle and removed all dietary and lifestyle estrogen one by one. The first thing I did was quit alcohol. I was only drinking 2-3 glasses of wine a week. I didn't realize that alcohol was impacting my health until I quit. Within 2 months of quitting, I was symptom-free, and I felt like myself again - well-rested, sharp, energetic, and leaner. So I began studying the effects of alcohol on perimenopause and aging.

The Unsung Hero

When it comes to perimenopause, there is one organ that needs our primary attention, the liver. This incredible organ is responsible for over 500 different functions in our body. During perimenopause, our liver function actually decreases by_1% per year[4]. It is crucial to protect this vital organ and prevent it from becoming overburdened in order to stave off

News-Medical - What is Perimenopause: https://www.news-medical.net/health/What-is-Perimenopause.aspx#:~:text=date%20is%20difficult.-,Perimenopause%20and%20estrogen,and%20fluctuate%20much%20more%20widely.
4. World Journal of Gastroenterology: https://www.ncbi.nlm.nih.gov/pmc/articles/PMC4491951/pdf/WJG-21-7613.pdf

diabetes, body fat, and poor health as we age.

A healthy liver regulates blood sugar and processes fats and toxins easily, yielding a high-functioning metabolism that efficiently converts nourishment into energy. When the liver is overburdened, it creates more fat and stores the toxins in the fat. Signs of an overburdened liver overlap perimenopause symptoms such as irritability, headaches, itchy skin, fatigue, brain fog, insomnia, weight gain, and constipation. Other signs that the liver is overworked include nausea, bruising, swollen ankles, and skin pigmentation.

When you drink alcohol, all of your liver functions are put on hold while your liver prioritizes detoxing the booze, which it perceives as poison. Instead of providing energy, the glucose and fat from your food are stored as body fat. In addition, your body doesn't absorb the nutrients, essential fatty acids, and fat-soluble vitamins it needs from your diet. You are further robbed when you drink because the liver uses your B vitamins to detox the alcohol.

One of the important functions your liver performs in perimenopause is clearing excess estrogen from your body. When you drink alcohol, you impair your body's ability to do this. The estrogen is then reabsorbed in the body and is stored in your fat. More on this later.

Boozy broads on the rise

The statistics are alarming - over the past decade, the

prevalence of Alcohol Use Disorders (AUDs) has surged[5] significantly among women compared to men. As women go through perimenopause, hormonal changes can affect how their bodies metabolize alcohol, making them more susceptible to alcohol-related damage.

Not so relaxing after all

Ah, sleep – that elusive companion. Sleep disturbances are a hallmark of perimenopause, and alcohol can further exacerbate the problem. Although alcohol may help some fall asleep initially, it disrupts the REM phase of sleep, leading to overall poorer sleep quality. Prioritizing restful sleep becomes paramount in our quest for sanity, overall well-being, and long-term brain health.

Perimenopause can be a rollercoaster of emotions, with low mood and mood swings being common occurrences. If you are wondering why you feel so blue after a boozy night, it's because alcohol is a central nervous system depressant.

The Show Stopper

Drinking in perimenopause is dangerous because it increases our risk of cancer. Alcohol consumption is the third major modifiable cancer risk[6] factor and less than 1 drink a day[7] is associated with an increased cancer risk.

5. Consideration of sex and gender differences in addiction medication response: https://bsd.biomedcentral.com/articles/10.1186/s13293-022-00441-3#:~:text=Over%20the%20past%2010%20years,consequences%20when%20compared%20to%20males
6. American Cancer Society: https://acsjournals.onlinelibrary.wiley.com/doi/10.3322/caac.21591
7. CDC - Facts about moderate drinking: https://www.cdc.gov/alcohol/fact-sheets/moderate-drinking.htm#:~:text=Alcohol%20has%20been%20found%20to,drink%20in%20a%20day

Alcohol is also estrogenic, meaning that it increases estrogen in our bodies. There is solid scientific evidence that higher levels of estrogen due to alcohol are associated with hormone-dependent breast cancer[8]. Many women are already experiencing higher levels of estrogen in perimenopause.

When we add alcohol to the mix, it places an extraordinary burden on our liver and allows that excess estrogen to recirculate and store in our body. It's a ticking time bomb. In addition to breast cancer, high estrogen levels increase the risk of ovarian and uterine cancer.

The good news

The amazing liver is the only solid organ that can completely regenerate itself after partial surgical removal or chemical injury. As long as you don't have chronic liver disease, your body will create a completely new liver every 3 years. So it's not too late to change your mind about booze.

There's no shame in admitting that alcohol may be negatively impacting your quality of life. You're not alone. Life can genuinely improve when you decide to put down the drink. Aside from the health benefits of quitting alcohol, sobriety is your ticket to stepping into a stronger, more authentic version of yourself and there is no better time than now.

8.Pubmed - Alcohol intake and risk of breast cancer defined by estrogen: https://pubmed.ncbi.nlm.nih.gov/18067133/

Get the insights, resources and motivation you need to remove the mystery of Midlife & Make Menopause the Best Period of Your Life.

Notes page

Make menopause the best period of your life.

CHAPTER THREE
Acceptance, the powerful perimenopausal anxiety antidote
by Jo Jones

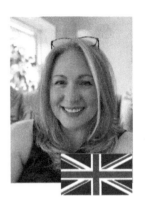

Bio: Jo Jones is The Peri Mind-Medicine Woman, an award-winning therapist, mindfulness teacher and perimenopause coach. She focuses on helping women to understand and recognise their thought processes, remove some of the scariness, dissolve shame gremlins, and hush their anxiety, to create a more self-compassionate and thriving version of themselves, on their empowered peri pathway.

Jo lives in the west country, near Bristol, UK with her partner, Jack, and their three over-affectionate dogs. She loves to bake bread, knit socks and is happiest with a large coffee, sunglasses on her head, walking in flip flops on a Cornwall beach.

Business: Hush TheraCoaching
Website: https://sleek.bio/johush

Anxiety is the unseen yet pervasive spectre that haunts the lives of many of us during perimenopause.

In fact, it's the most widely experienced symptom, sneakily woven into the tapestry of our fluctuating oestrogen levels, disrupting our stress hormone production, and challenging our emotional equilibrium.

Anxiety during perimenopause is not a statistic to me - it's a very personal experience. I understand it, not only because I've researched and studied it, but because I have lived it. However, amidst this bewilderingly chaotic dance of hormones, there is a powerful antidote that can significantly help soothe this anxiety: acceptance.

There was a time when acceptance felt like an alien concept to me, ridiculously out of reach. Each tide of hormonal change would bring waves of anxiety, sweeping me along, and in my resistance, I would flounder and go under. I was trapped in a spiralling cycle of railing. I couldn't believe that peri was happening to me. I hadn't joined the dots. At 47, I felt too young.

So, I had a big old rummage through my therapists' toolkit… blew the dust off my own stagnant unconscious mindset, and decided to experiment with the idea of acceptance, to lean into my peri experience rather than instinctively pushing it away.

It wasn't easy; our deep-seated survival instincts often seem insurmountable. However, as I took small steps toward accepting my situation, I noticed a shift. I began to conserve precious energy I previously wasted and instead I channelled it into finding solutions, opening my heart to new possibilities. I found a mental freedom I couldn't remember ever experiencing. My inner critic, once so loud, began to hush. Little by little.

Acceptance often gets misinterpreted and can cause inner friction when we begin to talk about it, I've found in my thousands of hours of client work… yet, by its true definition, is neither an experience, nor an act of passive resignation or endurance. It's not giving in, 'putting up with an awful situation' or grinning and bearing things. Just no.

It is a conscious choice, a nifty mindset tool that we can learn and choose to deploy, to powerfully disarm the threat and help us navigate the uncertain terrain of perimenopause. Far from signalling defeat, acceptance is an active and empowering, horn-tooting, strategy, to help us meet the reality of our present situation and make peace with it… as best we can, in any moment.

Which, gorgeous women, is ALL we can ever do.

Now, this might seem utterly counterintuitive to begin with. After all, our innate survival instincts, born from the ancient depths of our 'safety brain', our limbic system, resist perceived threats (and perimenopause can definitely feel threatening to our identity, relationship with our changing bodies, and our daily functioning).

"Who wants to go through perimenopause?! …almost

nobody! – We are designed to avoid and resist a dreaded experience"

It's a protective mechanism, an echo of our primitive selves that equates change and uncertainty with danger. Consequently, we RESIST in all kinds of ways. But in resisting, we unknowingly cultivate a breeding ground for anxiety.

"The only way out is through" - resistance in the context of perimenopause is quite a complex beast. What it actually does is burn up our resources, stifling our capacity for creative thinking and leaving us stuck in a dark, treacly vortex of frustration and fear. This resistance feeds fear, and cleverly hides the fact that any moment in which we experience an unpleasant or overwhelming thought or emotion, is simply a snapshot in time, not an unchanging reality. Most crucially, we are not stuck in that moment, but to move through it, we first need to come to a place of acceptance. Consciously, we know that humans are in a state of perpetual change throughout our entire lives... So why does this 'change' feel so very permanent and stuck? - Because we don't want it! We never signed up for it – and we can't know what will happen.

"Resistance is not your fault, by the way – it's nothing you are consciously doing wrong. Yet when we shine some loving acceptance light on it...it's pretty magical"

Acceptance involves acknowledging our current reality, as best we can, suspending judgement or dread. It means recognising that our experience of perimenopause isn't a punishment, an ending, or a sign of weakness. And instead, remembering that it's a natural phase on the ever-shifting continuum of womanhood. It requires us to be open, honest, and vulnerable, about our emotions, our changing bodies, and our needs. We can then soothe our emotional foundation enough to bring in a sense of curiosity, around what we are actually experiencing, rather than what we felt yesterday... or anticipate feeling tomorrow, or next week... or next year.

"Our primitive safety systems are designed to rake over everything awful we've ever felt, and project even more awfulness to come... why do they do that?"

Because this activity served us well, as cavepeople – it kept us safe. And the part of the brain that does this safe keeping is not intellectual, and in fact, hasn't had a software upgrade for about half a million years. It can't think of new ways of doing things. It keeps us entrenched in repeated patterns of behaviour to block, numb out and generally avoid... to resist! Our layers of physical and emotional safety nowadays are sophisticated, many, and varied; we have access to good information, we live in far safer conditions, we have resources like this, to help soothe, heal, and restore us. And maybe most importantly, we are talking about and sharing our peri experiences.

And once we do the acceptance thing? The load lifts. When we embrace acceptance, we pivot gracefully from stagnation to liberation, allowing ourselves the freedom to navigate our perimenopause pathway with greater ease. It's the first step in breaking the chain of resistance and the resulting anxiety, setting the stage for soothed and empowered problem-solving, and opening up a world of possibilities for healing and growth.

Once acceptance is embedded in our consciousness, we can layer in some glorious practices of self-compassion, further strengthening our emotional foundations. As we extend kindness towards ourselves, recognising our struggles without criticising ourselves for them, we create a soothing balm for the turbulent emotional soul seas that perimenopause can often stir.

This perimenopausal stage, while undoubtedly challenging at times, offers us a unique opportunity to reevaluate, reassess and reorientate ourselves on life's continuum. As we face our moment-by-moment experience, call out our fears with love, embrace acceptance, and extend compassion towards ourselves, we create a nurturing environment that paves the way for our personal peri evolution.

"In acceptance, we find resilience. We find the calm space to breathe, the space to be. We find the power to walk through perimenopause, not with trepidation, but with a sense of understanding and grace"

And remember, there's no need to face this alone. Join the community at HushPeri®, engage with resources, find understanding ears, and supportive voices who are walking the same path, dissolving anxiety, and transforming their lives, through the power of acceptance.

As we walk this pathway together, let's welcome a mantra of acceptance: "I am open to my experience, I acknowledge my emotions, and I embrace my peri pathway."

Because when we choose acceptance, we choose freedom, peace, and the power to navigate our way through perimenopause with dignity, courage, and above all self-compassion.

Now, I want to offer you a simple exercise to explore acceptance in your own perimenopausal journey, with my love, Jo x

Soothing light of Acceptance – HushPeri®

1. Settle in: Find a comfortable spot. Allow your body to settle and focus on your breath, just as it is – This is your safe space. Your breath is your constant anchor

2. Breathe, notice, and acknowledge: Close your eyes and take a deep breath in, hold for a beat, then exhale slowly. As you do this, acknowledge your current state. Are you feeling anxious? Calm? Irritated? Tired? Heavy? Content? – Accept those feelings without judgement and allow curiosity to take its place. This is your current reality. In this moment. Right now.

3. Visualise acceptance: Allow your experience to gently widen to just one or two recent experiences of peri that you'd like to soothe and move through...notice the body sensations that arise with those thoughts – With each inhale, visualise a soothing light of acceptance entering your body, filling you with wise understanding. Give the light a colour that represents calm, acceptance wisdom for you. Let it wash down through you... soothing whatever calls for your attention in the moment... and with every exhale, let things be... soften, soothe, allow.

4. Affirmation: Repeating to yourself, "I am open to accepting myself just as I am... and my experiences just as they are in this moment." "I am safe...all is well – I am moving on my peri pathway".

5. Reflect: After a few minutes of this exercise, reflect on how you feel. What's changed? I don't know whether the shift you feel will be subtle or profound, yet I do know that it will have an effect on your experience. This exercise is not about quick fixes; it's about gradual shifts towards acceptance.

Get more access to peri help with me in the HushPeri® Hub:

Journal prompt:

"If, for whatever reason, tomorrow, I began to feel more accepting of myself, exactly as I am, what would be the first thing I would be pleased to notice?"

"The wisdom you are growing into, is worth its weight in youth" – Unknown

CHAPTER FOUR
Burnout in midlife
by Nic Pendregaust

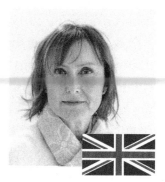

Bio: Helping peri-menopausal HR leaders feel lighter, brighter and in control and lead the way at work and at home. Nic is a qualified therapist with a counselling, coaching and hypnotherapy toolkit.

Business: Clarity Kent
Website: clarity-kent.co.uk

Embrace the midlife shifts. Slow down to speed up.

Yes, burnout & perimenopause are connected. So, if your stress glands were already overworked, during perimenopause they just cannot keep up with their usual responsibilities – the result is a hormonal rollercoaster as you find yourself running on adrenaline (probably with a large dose of caffeine & wine), which, put simply, is unsustainable.

Burnout can 'catch' us up in midlife. We are the 'sandwich generation' who have been juggling too much for too long without looking after ourselves and the reality being that our 40's & 50's can be the busiest time of our lives. You may be dealing with young adult children, caring for sick and/or elderly parents, a disconnected relationship, children at home or leaving home (empty nest syndrome), work pressures, financial challenges, supporting your partner at the same time as experiencing perimenopause symptoms; all varying forms of living loss in our hectic lives. All of this can lead to feelings of stress, overwhelm and ultimately, perimenopause burnout.

Acknowledging too, that we were all in the middle of a pandemic over the last few years but throw in the drop in oestrogen plus all the other 'stuff' us, midlife ladies are dealing with, and our risk of burnout is high.

With our hormones fluctuating, we need to rethink our energy highs and lows and start working with them rather than against them.

Burnout can be due to:
- running on adrenaline (empty) for years
- not addressing past trauma(s)
- lack of self-kindness & self-compassion
- people pleasing
- striving to achieve
- living in 'fight or flight' mode
- our nervous system being dysregulated
- being highly sensitive
- being an over giver
- putting others' needs before your own

- burning the candles at both ends (cue caffeine & wine)

There are several aspects to burnout, that we may not see coming. Here's a snapshot of what to look out for when your body is at *dis-ease*:

- **Mental burnout:** mental exhaustion, inability to focus, constant dissatisfaction with your work, and frequent headaches. Does this resonate if you are in a busy, high pressurised role and/or professional career?

- Then, there is **physical burnout:** physically exhausted, despite how much sleep you get, experiencing insomnia, chronic & frequent fatigue & increased dis-ease & sickness. Sound familiar?

- **Emotional burnout** can show up in us when we feel like we are a failure alongside apathy and loss of our mojo, constant self-doubt, experiencing depression, general feelings of hopelessness, increased anxiety, cynicism, or anger.

- And **social burnout** with sensory overload, an aversion to going out, feeling detached during engagement with others, and dreading social events.

How is burnout perceived by others around us? I wonder if most see it as a sign of weakness. Yet actually it is a sign of being strong (but for far too long). As women, we can experience this during menopause.

So, there are numerous reasons why people reach burnout, with different signs and symptoms during our midlife. We are all different and all cope in different ways too. When burnout happens, your body and mind are telling you "That's enough". Remember, our bodies give us clues. So we need to learn to listen to them.

Let's talk about some physiology basics. We become overstressed, our body releases cortisol and adrenaline. They surge in our body when we are under stress, playing a critical part in our health. Cortisol regulates vital functions, such as sleep, digestion, and your immune system. As part of your body's flight-or-fight-or-freeze response, it also keeps you alert and ready to face threats. That's why we produce more when stressed. And we certainly need to keep tabs on it when we are hormonal too! Lengthy periods of anxiety can lead to symptoms such as poor sleep, high blood pressure, headaches, weight gain and a compromised immune system leading to more infections. Cortisol also regulates your sleep-wake cycle. This is where we find a connection to burnout symptoms. When chronic stress elevates your cortisol levels, your sleep is put at risk.

Adrenal fatigue is when our adrenals 'burn out' from producing too much cortisol. causing hormone imbalances and symptoms. Again, adrenal fatigue can compound our distress in peri too – it's all connected!

Your body, however, doesn't ever 'burn out' or run out of hormones. If your system is constantly pumping out cortisol, even when threats are minor, your system becomes desensitised to stress. and that's when burnout symptoms can develop. It's crucial to interrupt the cycle of stress and put your health back on track.

So how can we feel calm in perimenopause and avoid, or at least minimise, burnout?

Firstly, acknowledge that you're stressed. Your body is giving you signals before you burn out. Recognise and acknowledge your feelings and symptoms. You may experience discomfort in doing this, yet your body is 'red flagging' you to take notice. Don't stick your head in the sand (aka Ostrich Syndrome).

Listen to your body: tune into what your body is telling you. You can change habits, prioritise yourself, manage your stress, be mindful and take time for YOU.

Look at what your triggers are that give rise to the stressful feelings. You can keep a diary of what your symptoms are and this may be helpful to join some dots so you can identify any patterns. Once you know what your anxiety triggers are, you can respond with actions to address them.

Self-care all the way: eat a healthy diet, stay away from sugar (as we know in menopause this increases inflammation in our body). Eat whole foods and a plant rich diet, balanced with protein, fat, fibre, and complex carbs: the so-called 'Mediterranean' diet.

Managing your time: Make a list of tasks you must do. Be realistic about what's achievable. Prioritise your list by deciding what's important and urgent.

Boundaries (those again). Saying No. Put boundaries in place so you can recharge your battery. Key to finding calm in your daily routine.

Get out into nature – See if you can get out into green space within the first 30 minutes of waking up. Being out in natural light can help to manage our melatonin level.

Get creative – This can be a great way of stimulating the brain and reducing stress. Colouring, drawing, painting, dancing all help us to feel calmer and happier.

Meditation & mindfulness – Research shows that these help to reduce stress. Try apps such as CALM, Headspace & Insight timer.

If you feel that 1-1 therapeutic coaching with me is for you, book a free informal zoom coffee chat with me here: calendly.com/clarity-kent & let's start a conversation.

Journal questions:

1.   Have you experienced burnout?

2.   What can you do differently to find calm in perimenopause and minimise and/or avoid burnout?

Embrace the power of midlife shift. Slow down to speed up.

CHAPTER FIVE
The Chinese medicine approach to resolving your symptoms naturally
by Andrea Marsh

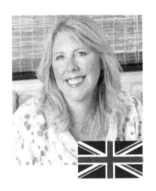

Bio: Andrea, a Chinese medicine and Shiatsu practitioner, deciphers and resolves menopause issues holistically. Her book "Understanding Your Menopause" offers proven natural solutions. Based in Cheltenham, UK, she's accompanied by Leela, her one-eyed Romanian rescue dog and feuding feline Tiddles. Andrea's passions include research, crafting, tennis, and mixing cocktails!

Business: Cotswold Menopause
Website: www.cotswoldmenopause.co.uk

"The hormonal transition is a stress in itself. You need to know this! A majority of what you're experiencing, especially in the perimenopause years leading up to menopause is caused by a depletion of nutrients to support your hormonal balance."

I'm not sure I would have got this far into my menopause transition, 52 and still very peri, without having the wisdom of Chinese medicine to guide me through. Helping me understand my changing body and very importantly what to do naturally to relieve my symptoms to feel energised and happy again!

At 46 I was really feeling it not knowing what it was; I just thought I was ageing and the M word wasn't even mentioned. Luckily though I was at a talk where it was mentioned and then bells in my head started ringing. I turned to my Chinese reference books as the symptoms were a confusion to me from a Chinese medicine point of view; the way they were all mixed together and could apparently happen at any time during the menopause transition. The only thing is though, your body works in a certain way so the mix of heat symptoms with Chinese medicine cold ones like anxiety and fatigue didn't make any sense to me; there is a biological order to symptom creation! I only had symptoms that were classed as cold ones, along with crying at everything, very low moods and my memory was shot; it wasn't a great time. Then I started asking my friends and clients, and they all said: I'm having a cold menopause too!

Enter Perimenopause! A time before you have the hot flushes and erratic/no periods; when symptoms are emerging but not the classic menopausal ones. Many of these are emotion-based like low moods and feeling unable to cope due to being easily overwhelmed.

The theory of Traditional Chinese Medicine (TCM) makes sense of how your body works under the covers. At that time, the known *34 symptoms of the menopause* just didn't make any sense to me from a TCM point of view, I had to work out how the symptoms were linked together, to solve my own list of ailments! It was confusing to me at first and took a couple of years to really get to grips with understanding it all; so how are you supposed to navigate the complexity of your changing body?

This is what drove me on to find results and help others that were in my situation or even worse.

COLD SYMPTOMS	HEAT SYMPTOMS
Fatigue	Night sweats
Anxiety	Irritability
Lower back ache	Mood swings
Low moods	Itchy skin
Dizziness	Dry skin
Heavy blood loss	Breast pain
Brain fog	Brittle nails
Memory issues	Vaginal dryness
Muscle/joint aches	Hot flushes
Incontinence	Headaches
Bad sleep 4/5am	Bad sleep 1/3 am

Using my TCM form of diagnosis I sorted out the jumble of symptoms into 2 groups: heat-related and cold-based ones. This means: what is the source within the body? For example, night sweats are heat-based indicating to me your liver needs help. Tiredness comes from the kidneys; fatigue is classed as cold and deficient. Excess symptoms like heat are quicker to resolve, and cold, deficient symptoms need something added into your body; nourishment.

Are all your perimenopause symptoms a deficiency?

Deficiency isn't openly talked about from a western point of view, but many women are vitamin B12 deficient and others have an underactive thyroid; just 2 examples. TCM delves deeper and looks to the organs/energies that are struggling to find a deficiency. The good news is that these can then be resolved so that symptoms dissipate or never happen. Supporting the thyroid before it goes wrong or ensuring your body never has a hot flush; these are obtainable from a TCM diagnosis and this also gives me the key to resolving your symptoms.

A majority of what you're experiencing, especially in the perimenopause years leading up to menopause (i.e. you have periods and symptoms) are caused by a depletion of nutrients to support your hormonal balance.

You may say – Oestrogen! But if you still have periods it's unlikely to be oestrogen; in fact you can have a dominance at this time that triggers symptoms. The hormone that is on decline during perimenopause is progesterone and it's also suppressed by cortisol, the stress hormone. Cortisol is released with adrenaline (exercise can cause more stress), so the key to helping your body in the long term is to manage stress in your life. However, to start feeling relief quickly, let's combat this depletion of nutrients that you have, as this is what is causing a majority of your symptoms.

You may have been putting up with fatigue, insomnia, aches, pains, anxiety, brain fog and a host of other symptoms without a hot flush in sight (and some of you may have flushes too!). I want you to know you can step in at any point, turn this around and *feel like YOU again*! This is where I was, a list of symptoms, feeling like a wreck but no hot flushes. Once I followed my own research, my symptoms started disappearing; anxiety almost overnight!

What is the deficiency that's causing your symptoms?

Answer: nutrients.

The hormonal transition is a *stress in itself*. You need to know this!

Your body needs fuel to live, more so as your hormones start to change; and that fuel is vitamins and minerals. Then add in the average stress levels of a 40+ woman and you just can't cope as well as you did previously. You may look back and reflect that you used to juggle complexities with ease and now you can't even remember what you're going to the fridge for! This is stress. It's taking its toll on your memory, mind and emotions; and stacking up in your body as physical symptoms.

Cortisol, the stress hormone, is released along with *adrenaline*. This isn't a bad thing, it's what's kept humans alive, but in the current modern lifestyle it's starting to be detrimental to your health and sanity.

Cortisol needs to be fed so that it can do its job effectively. If it can't get enough from your diet it starts leeching it from your body and you are feeling this as symptoms from joint aches to brain fog.

Feed *cortisol*, help it do its job and it dissipates, if you can plug this gap in your nutrient deficiency this then starts the rebalance of your hormones.

If your body is over producing *cortisol* it doesn't have the capacity to produce *progesterone* too. Once the *progesterone* in your ovaries starts declining the adrenals step in. The primary function of your adrenals though is to produce hormones to keep you safe; reproductive hormones are secondary. Quell your *cortisol* levels and your body can then produce more *progesterone*, in turn balancing out your high *oestrogen*; you'll be giving your body what it needs to heal; relieving an array of symptoms.

In TCM we say your body requires 3 things – good air, good food, good rest.

These are a few examples of how you can start to resolve your symptoms:

Add in fresh air – choose to walk in nature over the treadmill in the gym, for oxygenation of your body.

Add in good food – greenery first, then the rainbow of vegetables, fruits, nuts, seeds, wholegrains, protein too. Adding in supplements if you still have symptoms; feed your mind and body.

Add in quality rest – replenish your reserves; resting is revitalising! Combat stress with quality sleep rather than exercise. Look for mindfulness apps, meditation, Restorative Yoga, Qi Gong. Eastern exercise restores your energy; Western exercise, when overdone, depletes it.

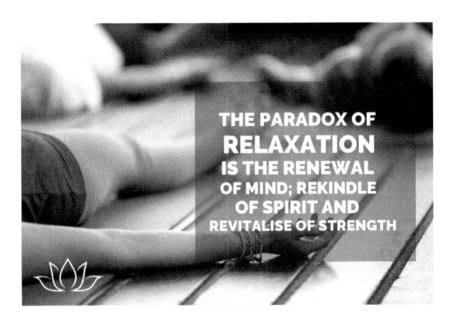

Find symptom relief with vitamins and minerals

Start with eating greenery every day of the week. Your gut needs greens, your liver needs greens. They are high in vitamins and minerals (more vitamin C than in fruit!) they are antioxidants and help clean your liver; this relieves heat symptoms. Don't forget hydration too, sipping room temperature water is the best way for your energy rejuvenation.

Due to current soil conditions you can't get enough nutrients from food to combat the levels of stress you're experiencing. If you have symptoms, you have stress. Even if you're at the stage of Hot flushes they stem from a prolonged period of stress in your body. If you've never had another symptom and only have hot flushes, you have physical stress in your body.

Think minerals over medication! You'll be on the right path to resolving your symptoms now and having better health in the coming years.

Stress strips the nutrients from your body to try and heal you. To help the healing cycle, give your body nutrients it needs.

Where do you get your nutrients from, if not food?

Start with plant-based supplements (and this is coming from someone who didn't take a supplement in their life!) - I've had a complete 180 turnaround as I feel so different since taking them. My symptoms went – anxiety, crying at everything, fatigue, muscle aches, brain fog. Every time something changes in my mind or body I go back to nutrients: what am I missing? What can help me? Herbals too; the right ones at the right time.

Why plant-based supplements?

Because they are made from vegetables; they are what your body can absorb and utilise. You may even find you're craving the likes of broccoli; this is your body asking for more! Plant-based supplements provide you with super amounts of vitamins like the B complex for energy and soothing your nervous system, plus your daily requirement of zinc and all the trace minerals.

Magnesium - you need this! It's the source for calming your nervous system, helping you sleep, reducing everything from anxiety to cramp. You. Need. Magnesium.

Herbal supplements are made from plants that have an energetic effect on your organs like your liver, blood and adrenals. If you need help cleansing your liver, herbals will do this. If you're anxious and exhausted, look to stress adaptogens, one that soothes you, calms the adrenal response and helps you regain your energy. Start with nutrients first though; pop petrol back in the tank before you add a turbo booster!

I want to empower you to have a great menopause; this means having a great life!

Perimenopause is worse for this generation because of the lifestyle we've been sucked into since childhood – work hard, go to the gym, carve up your sleep and eat convenience foods as you don't have time to cook. Then add in life situations; all this creating physical stress in your body, and making you feel like you're going mad or you can't cope. Increasing your nutrient intake is the magic pill you're looking for!

If I hadn't turned to my TCM books and taken the steps I've written about today, I would not have had the energy to pursue becoming a menopause specialist on top of my busy day to day Shiatsu practice. I want to show you how to get your vitality back too!

Ready to get started?

Andrea is the author of **Understanding Your Menopause: Tried and tested practical, natural solutions to alleviate your symptoms effectively.**

Love this chapter? Access the wisdom and direction necessary to understand and relieve both your physical and emotional symptoms with natural methods.

Check the QR code for my free guide: Inspiring Menopause!

Notes:

"Happiness is like a butterfly, the more you chase it, the more it will evade you, but if you notice the other things around you, it will gently come and sit on your shoulder."

CHAPTER SIX
Do You Trust Yourself With Food and Your Cravings?
by Tanya Stricek

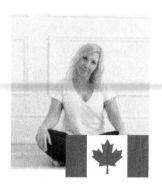

Bio: My name is Tanya and I'm a retired dental hygienist, turned non-diet nutritionist. I stopped dieting when I turned 50, while taking holistic nutrition and learning the practice of Mindful Eating. I did all this while my mom was dying. As I watched her decline I realized that I'd rather spend the rest of my years being IN my body with self love, and ease, and not stressing about my weight. Now I help women with menopause health in a way that helps them feel unconfined by food rules and aging.

Business: Tanya Stricek Non Diet Mindful Eating Nutritionist and Behaviour Coach
Website: www.tanyastricek.com

There is no shame in craving different foods

By the time you hit your 40's and 50's, and start moving through perimenopause and menopause, you're probably familiar with all kinds of cravings!

Emotions go up and down like a roller coaster at this stage of life, and many women note that they do more emotional eating. There is a consensus on the internet that the term emotional eating refers to the act of using food as a way to cope with, or soothe, emotions.

I've seen emotional eating defined as a common practice that many people engage in, without even realizing it. Yes, it is common. To emotionally eat, is to be human.

It is also a coping mechanism for some. How many of us have coped with stress by reaching for something to eat? We are living in a world where we are constantly exposed to stress, and stress can become chronic.

Stress is also a large part of the menopause transition and the act of chewing is a stress reliever! Mastication, or chewing, may reduce cortisol levels measured in plasma, and saliva. It reduces stress in the nervous system, particularly in a place called the hypothalamus[1]. This is a part of the nervous system that helps your body maintain homeostasis or balance. It signals your endocrine system and is part of the stress response.

Maybe you call your emotional eating a habit, and a "bad" habit, at that. It's a behavior that can bring on feelings of shame, guilt, and remorse. Why is that? It might have something to do with diet culture and body size. But is it inherently "bad"? I don't think so.

1. https://www.hindawi.com/journals/bmri/2015/876409/

Our society places great importance on thinness as part of beauty and health. Therefore emotional eating, overeating, eating without hunger, all get placed in a negative light. We internalize this eating as something flawed within us, and strive to control our eating with diets. Instead of placing emotional eating in this shameful light, let's look at the connections between emotions and food.

I always say that food, like a smile, is an almost universal communication tool. Food has a strong connection to our social ties, memories and emotions. Do you have childhood memories of certain foods that signified celebrations, days of the week, or that marked holidays? If those foods are associated with pleasant memories, then eating those foods may bring those feelings back, even for a little bit. This is one aspect of emotional eating.

When you think about the loss of a loved one, food can also be a connection. It's offered to support and nourish a grieving family. It soothes and nourishes you, in times of loss. Sympathy meals are a way to let someone know that you care, and are supporting them in times of sorrow.

It's a way of saying, "I care, and I don't know what to say."

Food is so much more than fuel. Food is memories, parties, gatherings, connecting with friends, or relaxing in the kitchen. Making meals is a creative outlet, and a relaxing activity for some. Foods are generational, handed down, passed on and food can be the building blocks of our story.

Food plays a role in so many settings, both joyous and sad, that it becomes very difficult to separate food and emotions. It is no wonder that we turn to food when we are feeling down or anxious.

When we eat, our brain releases feel good chemicals such as dopamine and serotonin, which are associated with pleasure and happiness. So, indulging in our favorite comfort foods can provide a temporary mood boost.

Conversely, this relief can be short-lived, and does not address the deeper roots of our emotions.

When I think of how I ate through the death of my fiance, so many years ago, I see a woman trying to fill a hole in a heart that can never be filled. At the biggest size of my life, I had just lost my partner, the father of my 22 month old. I wandered the kitchen at night, eating anything I could.

I needed to numb out. The trauma of his passing was too much. I also couldn't sleep. Insomnia made me hungry, and overwhelming grief made me hide in food.

I was in survival mode. Eating reminded me of my partner, the father of my child, who loved to cook. Eggs benedict, and chocolate fudge. French onion soup, and chocolate chip cookies. Mashed potatoes, and all kinds of sauces. Comfort foods. His mom's cabbage salad, that we can't find the recipe for anymore. You see, he was an emotional cook, and made things his mother and grandmother made. It made him feel connected.

If we were to look at food from a mindful eating perspective, emotional eating can be broken down into different types of hunger. According to Jan Chozen Bays, MD. the author of Mindful Eating, there are 9 types of hunger:

- Mouth Hunger
- Nose Hunger
- Eye Hunger
- Mind Hunger
- Cellular Hunger
- Heart Hunger
- Ear Hunger
- Touch Hunger
- Stomach Hunger

The topic of hunger itself is nuanced. If you are new to addressing your relationship to food, and gaining insight into your own emotional eating it might be simple just to separate physical hunger from emotional hunger.

Contrary to popular opinions, emotional eating in itself is not inherently bad or unhealthy. It is a normal and common behavior that many people engage in from time to time. It only becomes problematic when it becomes the primary coping mechanism for dealing with emotions. When it leads to a cycle of overeating, guilt, shame, remorse, and restricting your food, it can affect your mental well being.

If we look at emotional eating within the world of diet culture, we see food as the enemy, don't we? We tie emotional eating to weight gain, and the negativity of body size. This becomes increasingly difficult to navigate as we transition through perimenopause, and menopause, with the body and weight changes that many of us experience.

We have a hard time seeing that choosing to eat can be a form of self care. If you struggle with body image, this form of self care can turn into self hate. It's a vicious circle.

This begs the question, "Doesn't emotional eating impact our PHYSICAL health?" Emotional eating *can* have the *potential* to impact our physical health. This depends on our food selection, and frequency of consumption of certain types of foods. Consuming high-calorie, sugary, or fatty foods in excess may influence the risk of some health conditions such as fatty liver, blood sugar issues, and increased cardiovascular disease risk.

Additionally, the guilt associated with emotional eating may disrupt normal eating patterns, leading to bingeing and restriction. This can affect your nutrition quality, your digestion, elimination, and can walk the fuzzy line of an eating disorder.

It is important to note that emotional eating does not always have a significant impact on physical health.

Health is more than food. It is a combination of the social determinants of health, and includes many things that are not in our control! This includes race, genetics. socioeconomic status, working conditions, and childhood experiences. This topic goes way beyond what one chapter in a book can share.

The negative and positive impacts of emotional eating are not black and white. They are different for everyone. These impacts can extend to our mental well being and emotional health, too.

In one episode of the Fullness Podcast, I shared my kitchen cupboard story, where I feel my journey of emotional eating began. I had to let myself in after school, and I was very young. My mom was a single mom, and had to work. I came home to an empty house, without my mom or dad, and a cupboard full of food. Food became my companion. It quieted loneliness and rejection.

As I grew older, and became aware of how others viewed my body and its size, negative feelings about my eating patterns, low self esteem, and anxiousness about my looks, grew. This is where the desire to diet started in me. I berated myself for not being able to control myself when it came to food. I felt like a failure, and blamed my emotional eating for my size and shape.

How could I recognize that my emotional eating was a sign that there were unmet emotional needs that required attention? I was young, and didn't have the tools to do so.

I didn't acquire them until I turned 50. It's never too late to shift your mindset around food, weight, body image and age.

Shifting your perception of emotional eating, to a more balanced state with food, requires a combination of awareness, self-reflection, self-compassion, and mindful eating practices. It also requires patience with yourself. Let's look at some of these:

Self-awareness: Take the time to identify your emotional triggers for eating. Awareness is part of a Mindful Eating practice. Are you truly hungry? Are you feeling stressed, or another emotion, and want to reach for food? The key here is to JUST practice awareness and not change, as a first step. Eating triggers can include emotions, and also your environment, behavior and your own biology. Allow eating for comfort to be an option, and practice the next step, if you are able.

Self-compassion: Do you know how to be kind to yourself? Many of us do not. Understand that emotional eating is a common behavior and that it takes time to become aware of your habits around food. Treat yourself with compassion and avoid self-judgment or negative self-talk. I always say criticism never sparks change, but curiosity can. So can self-compassion.

Your wise mind: This is also a part of a mindful eating practice, where you combine the rational thinking part of your mind and the emotional part of your mind, to come to a place where you can make wise decisions about what YOU need in your food life. This way of thinking can help you with any health choice and decisions about your needs!

Staying present: Paying attention to the present moment, while eating, can bring you pleasure and satisfaction with your food, instead of guilt and shame. This engages your body cues and helps you practice eating for body signals, instead of what a diet dictates. Slow down, engage your senses, and truly experience the taste, texture, and aroma of your food. This can help you become more attuned to your body's hunger and fullness cues. It might also help you feel more satisfied, and have less cravings.

These are some foundations of mindful eating.

Growing up with diet culture has blocked our ability to listen to our body. Instead of tuning in to our needs, we ignore them. Emotions are stuffed down, along with the food. We cut off our ability to recognize hunger, and fullness, and even our ability to feel satisfied without food.

Diet culture has us using tricks to cut off hunger, like drinking water and coffee to suppress hunger signals. This can have lasting effects into menopause, as we may be missing key nutrients and minerals that feed bone health, brain health and more. Lack of food is perceived as a stressor by the brain, and this can also affect your journey through perimenopause.

What if we accepted right now that emotional eating is part of our human experience here? We all find ways to cope. This is called being human.

Life, and cake, were meant for savoring.

This is not intended as medical or mental health advice. Please seek help from a licensed care practitioner for any health concern or if you suspect you have an eating disorder.

If you'd like to hear more, meet me on YouTube!

Journal prompts:

Take time to identify your triggers for emotional eating.

How can you be kind to yourself today?

What can you do to be present right now?

CHAPTER SEVEN
Death – The Final Taboo
by Chloe Middleton

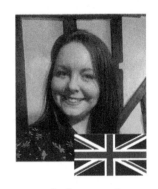

Bio: Chloe is a self-employed civil celebrant and also works as a funeral director for Rosedale Funeral Home across Suffolk. She lives in Bungay with her partner, Wayne and two sons, Logan and Jim. As well as spending time with family and friends, she enjoys wine (very much!), good books and long walks at the coast.

Business: CM Civil Celebrant
Website: cm-civilcelebrant.co.uk

Having worked in palliative care when I first left school and then in the funeral industry for the last fifteen years, initially as a funeral director and more recently in the role of a celebrant conducting funeral services, it has always been glaringly apparent to me how much we struggle as a society with the concept of death and dying. Especially in comparison to other cultures, we as British citizens tend to shy away from the only certain thing any of us have in our lives. The question this poses with regards to perimenopause and indeed menopause itself is…..would we embrace the changes to our bodies as a natural progression through life, if the idea of aging and ultimately our own mortality wasn't such a taboo subject?

We live in a society where in general death is not an open discussion point. I have often found, even with people close to me, if they are questioned about their own funeral wishes for example, then this is a talking point 'for another day.' We would prefer to ignore the inevitability of death and perhaps naively attempt to believe that life goes on forever and with that, our unadulterated youth.

Over time, death has become a subject that is shrouded in fear of the unknown. This is particularly true for women who tend to think of all eventualities on numerous different levels, the what ifs, buts and maybes that could potentially happen in the event of their own death. Who will pay the bills? Who will do the shopping? And in some instances, who will be there for the children?

This fear of the unknown is the same for women who begin to show symptoms of perimenopause and these changes in their bodies ultimately mean they are getting ever closer to being 'old' and therefore death itself. Similarly, a deep-rooted fear of death can be a real symptom associated with perimenopause and with these uncontrollable changes taking places in their bodies, some women have reported feeling as if they were about to die. These feelings bring fear, and ultimately a fear of death itself to the forefront of their mind, which may otherwise have remained in the background of their conscious.

This fear needs to be recognised and acknowledged to the women suffering from it. They also need to be reassured that they are not alone and for some as scary as it may be at the time, it is a real symptom of this natural process.

On a daily basis, we are exposed to images of 'the perfect woman' through the media. These are often young women, who may have been photo edited or enhanced with plastic surgery or similar. At a time when we are beginning to acknowledge that perimenopause may begin for some women as early as their mid-thirties, this can be extremely destructive to the mental health and body images of those whose bodies are changing (yet again) in the course of the life of a woman.

We can see a grief process itself in many women who are beginning to show symptoms of perimenopause. Many of the stages of grief (similar to those that may be experienced upon losing a loved one) may be presented by some women, due to them grieving the assumed loss of their youth. Depression and anxiety, anger at the uncontrollable nature of the situation, guilt about how they may have dealt with things in their lives and perhaps the most destructive of all human emotions, the ability to see things with hindsight. This emotion provides us as humans with nothing but negativity and as a result a feeling of failure. Being able to see what and how you would have done things differently given a chance but (which we already consciously know) with no possible ability to go back and change certain outcomes.

Hormones, or a lack of them, can wreak havoc with our ability to see things clearly and in an unbiased way. This is made ever more difficult by the fact that society continually reiterates that the ultimate perfection is to remain young at all costs but due to this many people are not aware of the privilege of aging itself. Aging is a process that so many are denied as their lives have been cut short prematurely. Everybody reading this has had the privilege of being young but far fewer gain the privilege of growing old, and it is a privilege.

So, what if we turned the concept around and viewed perimenopause as something to reassure us that we are going through yet another natural process of life and being alive? If we gain the ability to do this, then perhaps the concept of death itself becomes much less scary?

Ultimately, the finality of death will come to each and every one of us and so while we are still here, however challenging these changes may be, let's take the time to embrace each day and even on the days when it's overwhelming (which at times it will be) take time for some self care and positive thought reflection. We all have the ability to at least attempt to turn anything we may see as negative into a positive, the perspective is ours and we own the right to change it. We are fortunate that through books like this and the knowledge regarding perimenopause that we are gaining as women on a daily basis, we are more informed and supported now than we have ever been before. We have come so far from the generations before us who still faced these challenges but did so usually alone as the subject of menopause itself was so taboo.

So, to conclude, let's join together to be grateful for other women to whom we can look to for guidance, inspiration and a different perspective, the fact that we are fortunate enough to experience this process and ultimately take the fear out of our inevitable demise and enjoy the opportunities life brings whilst we are able to.

Contact Chloe on chloe@cm-civilcelebrant.co.uk

Journal prompts:

Where do I stand from my personal perspective with the prospect of aging and my own mortality?

What feelings can I acknowledge?

How do my feelings relate to perimenopause and are they different now to how I felt before?

What action can I take to validate my feelings and move forward?

CHAPTER EIGHT
Is it Time to Call a Divorce Lawyer?
by Rebecca Franklin

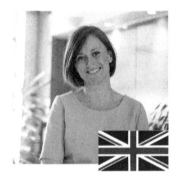

Bio: I'm a Family Lawyer of almost 30 years experience. I have a friendly, straight talking attitude to help my clients at a difficult time. I'm here to help my client's not fuel the fire!

Business: working with Woolley & Co
Website: www.family-lawfirm.co.uk

I have been practising as a family lawyer for almost thirty years. Notwithstanding the length of time I have been carrying out my work, there is never a dull moment and two days are never the same.

I've learnt that there is no one size fits all approach and every client, and their case is unique. It is important to me that anyone contemplating a separation is fully informed as to all of their options before they make that giant step. Knowledge is power at such a difficult time, and it is important that if someone is contemplating a separation that they find out first where they will stand afterwards from a legal and financial perspective.

I am going to focus the remainder of this chapter on giving advice to someone who is married. Obviously, this guidance would change if I were dealing with an unmarried couple.

What is a divorce?

Obvious as this may seem, a divorce is the legal process that ends your marriage. It is a positive that from April 2022 we had a change in law, and we now have a "no fault" divorce system. You now do not need to blame your spouse for the breakdown of your marriage to be able to apply for a divorce. Nor do you have to have been separated for a particular length of time before you can ask for a divorce – as you did under the old rules.

The only criteria now for a divorce (in England and Wales) is that you must have been married for at least one year.

The "downside" to the new divorce procedure is it takes much longer than the old one. Whereas under the old "blame" system a divorce would take around three to four months, now, it takes around seven to eight months.

As much as I dislike the longer process, we are stuck with it and there are no loopholes to shorten the process.

It is now nigh on impossible for your spouse to defend a divorce under the new system and you will not physically need to attend Court, the process is all dealt with online.

The divorce itself goes through a set timetable and is a fixed procedure. We spend most of our time dealing with any children and financial issues.

Children

The Court's attitude towards children is that these are your children, you decide how they divide their care between you. The Judges do not favour mothers - a very common misconception - and both parents are very much treated and viewed as equals in the eyes of the Court. Whilst I accept that in the mid-nighties (when I first started practice) fathers often felt that they were having to beg to see their children, it is a completely different landscape now and "sharing" is very much the buzzword of the moment.

Obviously, your children are not an object for you to divide, but I often find that the Courts agree that both parents should spend time with the children midweek – it is no longer the case that one parent can only expect to see their children at weekends. We live in a modern age where parents often have complicated shift patterns. This coupled with all of the afterschool clubs and extracurricular activities our kids' carryout nowadays, often make for some very complicated patterns for contact indeed – but the Court will take all of this into account.

The Courts adopt a strict "no order" principle about children and the Court will not get involved unless there is an issue. It is a common misconception that separating couples believe they must go to Court to get an order about their children – this is not the case.

Finances

The starting point for the Court is to divide all assets equally. The Court will move away from equality if there is a justification for it, considering the income that each party has, the ages of any relevant children etc.

The simplest way for me to explain this is that a family has been used to sharing one property and pooling resources. On divorce the task for the Court is to somehow divide the money so that both parties can both move on, each having a roof over their head enough money to put food on the table. If this can be achieved by simply dividing the assets equally, then this is what will be done. If one party needs to receive more than half to achieve this –that is the approach the Court will take.

The Court does not solely look at any assets or debts that a couple has, the Judge also needs to have evidence to show how much money a person would need to either rent/buy a new property and if a party wanted to buy a new property, they would need to produce evidence of the mortgage they could obtain to help with the purchase.

The Court can divide or transfer ownership in property,

money in pensions, bank accounts, shares etc. No assets are off limits, even those in other countries. Any assets you own anywhere in the world need to be disclosed.

Whilst I have mentioned in this section the approach the Court takes to the division of assets; the reality is that we try to avoid going to a Judge to decide a case like the plague!

If your case goes to a Judge to decide, then you can expect substantial legal fees and long delays on the part of the Court. It is not uncommon for a Judge to take a year to decide a financial case. It is therefore much better if you can negotiate a settlement between lawyers who will be able to guide you on what a Judge is likely to do, and you can be certain that you are achieving a fair settlement based on the parameters of the orders that the Judge would be likely to make.

If you can agree your case outside of Court, then the lawyers will draft up the paperwork for you to make this agreement legal and your settlement terms are then sent into the Judge to approve – again without the need to physically attend a Court hearing.

Obviously negotiating through solicitors can also be very time consuming and expensive and so my first advice to clients is that they instead mediate to try to negotiate a settlement without relying on lawyers. Family mediation is an excellent tool for a separating couple. A skilled and independent mediator will help you both explore your options, in terms of any children and financial issues. If you can agree at mediation, you would then only be coming back to the lawyers to help make your financial agreement legal.

This is going to reduce the amount of costs you are going to pay significantly. I have no qualms in saying that mediators are often cheaper than lawyers and if you instruct one mediator between you, rather than a lawyer each – there is a saving to be had automatically!

Advice to a friend

If you are considering a separation, it is important you speak to someone experienced who approaches family law in a constructive and transparent way. I would not want to speak to somebody and be sold a dream that I am going to get an amazing settlement and everything will be great with no problems!

The reality is that divorce, financial or children proceedings are very time consuming and can be very expensive. The expense is not only financial but also worse an emotional one. Whatever your views on your spouse are at the time of separation, you each need to be able to move on and it is not about trying to secure your pound of flesh. Family law in real life is not dealt with in the same way as it is in TV shows or movies.

No matter how hurt you are and no matter how much you want to blame your spouse (even if they deserve it) our legal system is not a punitive one and you can expect to hear phrases that include the words "equality", "sharing" and "needs". If you have children together you are going to have to co-parent those children, arguably for the rest of your lives. No matter how old children become, they all still need their parents, and if they decide to get married themselves, have children and so on, there are lots of occasions that you and your spouse will need to attend together.

Take your time, there is no rush to jump in with both feet and make a decision. Marriage counselling can be an excellent tool and something I would highly recommend.

Knowledge is power! Email me at Rebecca.Franklin@family-lawfirm.co.uk to find out where you stand rather than second guessing.

Notes:

CHAPTER NINE
Discover Your Hormone Hero: How DUTCH Testing Can Transform Your Perimenopause Journey
by Eleanor Duelley

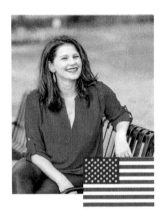

Bio: I'm passionate about helping women achieve vibrant balance through functional testing, therapeutic supplements, and transformative nutrition, all working together to up-level their lives from within.

Business: Eleanor Duelley Nutrition
Website: http://www.nourishingnutrition.net/
Instagram: https://www.instagram.com/holistic.hormone.specialist

In the midst of the whirlwind that is life, it's easy for women in their middle years to feel like they're losing control of their bodies and vitality. If you're like many of us, you've experienced the frustration of being told to rely on medications and diets that just don't seem to work. It's time for a change – a real, lasting change that doesn't mask symptoms but gets to the root of the issue. Welcome to a journey where you're not just a passive observer of your health, but an empowered driver of your well-being.

The Unveiling of Hidden Insights

Picture this: you're at a crossroads, feeling exhausted, carrying the weight of uninvited pounds, and tired of the constant battle with burnout. Traditional medical solutions seem to fall short, leaving you wondering if there's a way out of this cycle. It's here that we introduce a game-changer – the invaluable practice of getting your hormones tested. This isn't just about tracking numbers; it's about unlocking the doors to your body's intricate regulatory systems, shedding light on potential imbalances before they take hold, and paving the way for informed decisions that will redefine your health and well-being.

Unlike generic health assessments, hormone testing offers a unique window into the subtle symphony of your body's rhythms and cycles. It's a tool that pierces through the surface, allowing you to comprehend the nuanced interplay of physiological and hormonal dynamics driving your experiences. After all, the key to transformation is understanding, and hormone testing provides the roadmap to that understanding.

Beyond the Snapshots: The Power of DUTCH Testing

Now, let's talk about DUTCH testing – the beacon of clarity in the world of hormone assessment. Unlike conventional blood work that only captures a single snapshot of hormone levels, DUTCH testing unfolds over a 24-hour period, capturing the ebb and flow of your hormones. This comprehensive approach reveals insights into hormone production, metabolism, and imbalances that other methods may miss. Say goodbye to incomplete pictures and hello to a complete understanding of your body's hormonal landscape.

DUTCH testing transcends the superficial and dives deep into the very fabric of your hormonal health. It delves into hormone metabolites, unearthing essential information about how your body processes hormones. This is where the true magic happens – understanding the why behind imbalances and addressing the root causes that conventional testing might overlook.

You wake up one morning, feeling like you barely slept despite hitting the pillow early. You've got those stubborn pounds that seem to cling no matter what you do, and your energy is in a constant state of "meh." Your chin hair is making an appearance at the least opportune times, and your once vibrant libido is giving you the cold shoulder. And the most frustrating part? Conventional wisdom and advice just aren't cutting it.

Enter the DUTCH test. This powerhouse of a test goes beyond the basics. It's not just about checking off a few hormone levels – it's about getting the full scoop on your hormonal story. Picture it as a detective, uncovering clues to why you're feeling the way you are.

First up, sleep habits. Remember that night where you tossed and turned? DUTCH testing can reveal the secret conversations happening between your sleep hormones – cortisol and melatonin. Are they working together like a well-oiled machine, or is there a bit of a squabble going on, causing those restless nights?

Now, let's talk adrenal output. Those little glands play a huge role in your energy and stress response. DUTCH testing doesn't just show you how much cortisol you're producing; it gives you a glimpse into how your adrenals are pumping throughout the day. This is like looking at your stress levels on a graph – a real eye-opener.

And estrogen dominance? Oh boy, that's where things get really interesting. DUTCH testing doesn't just tell you if you have high estrogen; it shows you how your body is processing and breaking it down. You might have heard about those pathways – the good and the not-so-good ones. Well, this test puts them under the spotlight. Is your estrogen being metabolized into helpful, friendly compounds or those not-so-friendly ones that can mess with your balance? This can be a game-changer for those pesky symptoms like chin hair and weight loss resistance.

It's actually that good.... DUTCH testing is like your hormone whisperer. It looks at androgen symptoms – think mood swings, acne, and that elusive libido. It dives into your cortisol pattern, showing you if your stress response is balanced or if it's sending your hormones into a tailspin. It even checks in on your progesterone, that calming hormone that often takes a backseat to estrogen. Are you producing enough to keep things in check?

Now, here's the real magic – DUTCH testing validates what you're feeling. You're not crazy; your symptoms are real, and they have reasons. That chin hair, those mood swings, the weight loss resistance – they're not just in your head. They're signals, and the DUTCH test helps translate them. It's like having a heart-to-heart chat with your body, and it's finally getting the chance to speak up.

So, why does all of this matter? Because knowing is power. When you have the puzzle pieces, you can put them together and see the bigger picture. You're not blindly trying solutions; you're choosing the right path based on concrete information. It's like having a treasure map to your health and well-being.
By diving into your hormonal landscape, we're not just guessing. We're making informed decisions based on what your body is telling us. It's about finding the root causes, addressing them head-on, and creating a plan that's tailored to you. No more generic advice or one-size-fits-all solutions – this is about you, your unique story, and your individual needs.

And that's where I come in. As your Holistic Hormone Specialist, I'm here to be your partner in this journey. I've been in your shoes – tired of being told to settle for less, frustrated by the lack of solutions that truly resonate. Let's connect and have a heart-to-heart chat. We'll go over your

DUTCH test results, piece together your hormonal puzzle, and create a roadmap that's all about you. No more gaslighting, no more uncertainty – just a clear path to reclaiming your vitality.

The Empowerment of Knowledge

Empowerment lies at the heart of your journey. Armed with the insights from DUTCH testing, you're no longer at the mercy of surface-level solutions. I curate targeted protocols for natural healing, based on your unique results, using healing supplements and practical nutritional practices. What's even more astounding is that most women experience significant results by simply adjusting daily habits they didn't even realize were impacting their hormones.

Here are five easy actions you can start implementing today:

- Reduce Toxic Exposure: Swap chemical-laden cleaning products for natural alternatives to minimize endocrine-disrupting compounds in your environment. You can do this by starting to read the labels and check out what the ingredients actually contain.

- Mindful Food Storage: Opt for glass or stainless steel containers instead of plastic to avoid hormone-disrupting chemicals (plastics that break down when heated) leaching into your food.

- Clean Beauty Choices: Choose personal care products free

from parabens, phthalates, and synthetic fragrances to support your hormonal balance. This is crucial to allowing your body to naturally start detoxing better.

- Embrace Organic: Prioritize organic foods to reduce your exposure to pesticides and potential hormone-disrupting chemicals. These chemicals in your food are so harmful!

- Stress Relief: Engage in daily stress-relief practices like mindful breathing to support a balanced hormonal environment. I can help you figure out the best practices for you, as your experiences are unique and not like everyone else's.

Your Path to Renewed Vitality

Remember, this isn't just about health – it's about honoring your body, embracing your journey, and stepping into your power. Let's rewrite your story, together. Your vibrant, energized self is waiting, and I'm here to guide you every step of the way.

If you're ready for a paradigm shift, I'm here to guide you. As a Holistic Hormone Specialist, I understand your journey intimately. I've been where you are – frustrated with the lack of understanding, tired of being offered temporary fixes, and yearning for sustainable solutions. Let's take the reins together. In our first video conversation, we'll explore how you can naturally restore harmony to your hormones. Tailored testing, healing supplements, and manageable daily habits will pave your path to rejuvenation – not just for today, but for the years ahead.

This is your invitation to embrace health on your terms, to honor your body, and to embrace the passage of time with resilience and grace. The time for change is now. Let's make this journey together – your holistic hormone healing awaits.

Sign up for a free 20 min call to discuss how you can get testing now:

Notes:

CHAPTER TEN
What To Eat In Perimenopause
by Helen Jones

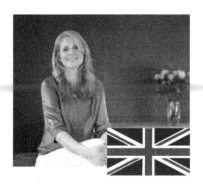

Bio: Hi, I'm Helen. I'm a BANT and CNHC registered Nutritional Therapist and an ILM Accredited Wellbeing Coach. I specialise in supporting women through perimenopause and menopause, helping them to take control of their health and hormones, so they feel energised, vibrant and more like themselves again.

I offer a range of 1:1 and group programmes which combine nutrition, lifestyle and supplement therapy, along with health and mindset coaching, to help you easily and successfully embed dietary and lifestyle habits that will get you back to feeling your best.

Business: Helen Jones Nutrition
Website: www.helenjonesnutrition.com

"Let food be thy medicine and medicine be thy food" Hippocrates

The power of food

Food is powerful. It can literally change the way we think, feel and look. It can change the way our bodies work and the likelihood of us getting sick. It can tell our bodies whether to burn or store fat, increase or decrease our energy, alter our mood, fuel or dampen inflammation, and switch genes for disease on or off.

In perimenopause, food can make a huge difference to how you experience this time of life. Sure, it's not a cure-all for everything, but the right nutrition can go a long way in reducing symptoms like fatigue, energy fluctuations, mood swings, anxiety, depression, weight changes, bloating, joint pain, migraines and even hot flushes.

And it's not just about the here and now. What we put on our plate can also have a profound impact on our *future* health, helping to reduce the risk of osteoporosis, heart disease, diabetes, depression, and obesity, which we know are all linked to the hormonal changes of perimenopause and menopause.

If there is any one time to get on top of your nutrition, it is during perimenopause. If you don't, your experience of perimenopause could be much worse and your risk of health problems in the future is likely to be increased.

Time to ditch the diet

Before we go into the specifics of what to eat in perimenopause, I want to make one very important point:

Making changes to the way you eat during perimenopause is NOT about 'dieting' and calorie restriction.

I know it can be tempting to go on a crash diet if we want to shed a bit of perimenopausal weight, however this can be detrimental to our health and even counterproductive. A very low-calorie diet puts our body into survival mode (think stress hormones), slows down our already declining metabolism and tells our body to hold onto fat reserves. Our undernourished, deprived body is left feeling even more tired, miserable and craving calories. So, guess what? We give up and go back to our normal diet. However, because our metabolism has slowed down so much, we quickly gain any weight we may have lost and more. Our precious adrenals, thyroid and blood sugar are also worse off for the experience which can exacerbate many other symptoms we may be experiencing during this time.

Perimenopause then, is the time to stop thinking about food as just numbers and say goodbye to those low-calorie diets. Now is the time to really start thinking about food as information and nourishment for your body, and shift your mindset to eating for hormone balance, bone health and metabolic regulation.

Just to really hammer this point home, let's think about the humble avocado versus a low-calorie cereal bar. Now I know many women fear the avocado because of the 200-300 calories they contain (thank you Weight Watchers and Slimming World!). However, avocado provides an abundance of healthy fats, fibre, vitamins and minerals, that nourish your hormones, keep your blood sugar stable, reduce cravings, mood and energy crashes and actually tell your body to burn fat. A 100-calorie cereal bar on the other hand, often has very little nutrition, contains refined carbohydrates, sugars and unhealthy fats that play havoc with our hormones, spike blood sugar, tell our body to store fat and results in cravings, mood and energy crashes shortly after. Can you see which one would be more helpful to you during perimenopause?

General Dietary Guidelines for Perimenopause:

So, now we are clear on the food as information and nourishment for our body, let's dive into some general guidelines for eating during perimenopause that will help mitigate symptoms and reduce the risk of future health issues.

Mediterranean Diet: While there's no one-size-fits-all diet for perimenopause, the Mediterranean diet comes closest to a universally beneficial style of eating. This revolves around unprocessed whole foods, including fruits, vegetables, beans, lentils, nuts, seeds, wholegrains, healthy fats like extra virgin olive oil and a moderate amount of fish, dairy and lean meat. Extensively researched, this anti-inflammatory, high fibre, low-sugar diet offers benefits across all areas of health; from bone and metabolic health to mood and cognition.

Embrace Low Glycaemic Load (GL) Foods: The glycaemic load refers to a food's effect on blood sugar. A high GL food is one with a high sugar or carbohydrate content that enters the bloodstream quickly (e.g. white bread, rice, pasta, cakes, biscuits, sweets etc). This sharp blood sugar spike is quickly followed by a crash, which leads to a dip in energy and mood, and sugar cravings. Because our blood sugar regulation can get a bit wobbly anyway during perimenopause, it's more important than ever to adopt a low GL way of eating. That is, consuming foods that release energy slowly and help keep blood sugar more stable. Not only will this help to reduce energy crashes, mood swings and sugar cravings (and prevent unwanted weight gain), it will help reduce the risk of diseases related to higher blood sugar such as heart disease, Type 2 Diabetes and dementia.

Low GL foods include certain fruits (e.g. berries, apples, citrus), vegetables, beans, pulses, lean meats, fish, eggs, nuts, and seeds. There are lots of books and resources online which help you get your head round the low GL way of eating, and I recommend you check these out if needed.

Prioritise Protein: Protein is a superhero nutrient during perimenopause. It supports lean muscle mass, boosts your metabolism, slows down the release of sugar into the blood, increases satiety hormones and reduces cravings. It's also essential for hormone production and detoxification. Good sources include organic meat, fish, dairy, eggs, nuts, seeds, beans, lentils, quinoa and organic tofu.

Each person's needs for protein varies depending on age, body size, activity level, and eating pattern, but generally I would recommend women in perimenopause aim for 20-30 grams of protein (or a palm-sized portion) at every meal. Eating protein at breakfast is particularly important and can make a huge difference to your energy levels and mood for the rest of the day. Eggs, natural yoghurt with nuts and seeds, or a green protein smoothie are great protein options for breakfast.

Make Fat Your Friend: We have been brought up to believe all fats are bad, however this couldn't be further from the truth! Healthy fats such as nuts, seeds, olives, avocado, oily fish, organic dairy, eggs, grass-fed meat, olive oil and coconut oil are essential for both mental and physical health. Not only are they required for hormone production, transport and storage, but they reduce inflammation (think joint pain), support the immune system, stabilise blood sugar, promote satiety, minimise cravings, reduce anxiety and depression and may even help with symptoms such as hot flashes, night sweats and sleep disturbances.

To ensure you get enough of the essential omega-3 fats, I would recommend eating oily fish (e.g. salmon, mackerel, sardines) 2-3 times a week, or supplement with a good quality Omega 3 Fish Oil or Algae oil if you are vegetarian/vegan.

Veg Out: Vegetables are nutritional powerhouses, and they deserve a prominent place on your plate during perimenopause. They are packed full of antioxidants, vitamins and minerals as well as fibre, which helps with digestion, gut health and blood sugar balance. Aim to fill at least half your plate with a colourful assortment of vegetables. Go for variety and try to eat the rainbow every day, as all the different colours have different nutrients. Don't forget the cruciferous veg like broccoli, cabbage, cauliflower, kale, and Brussels sprouts. They contain compounds that support liver detoxification and the clearance of excess oestrogen, and 1-2 portions of these a day may help alleviate symptoms like PMS, breast tenderness and bloating.

Calcium and Vitamin D3: Declining oestrogen means your bones have a harder time retaining calcium, which puts you at risk for weak and brittle bones and conditions such as osteopenia or osteoporosis or increased fractures. We therefore need to ensure a steady supply of calcium-rich foods in our diet, like almonds, leafy greens, sardines and pilchards, full-fat dairy, fortified plant milk, kale, broccoli or calcium-set tofu. Vitamin D3 is essential to calcium absorption, so make sure you get enough sunlight or consider supplementation.

Water: The benefits of water are massively underrated! Every cell in our body needs water, it transports hormones and vital nutrients, facilitates digestion and detoxification, helps maintain skin elasticity, supports weight management and aids cognitive function and mental clarity. Adequate water intake can also help relieve common perimenopausal symptoms like bloating, water retention, hot flashes, and headaches. My advice is to aim for 2 litres (3.5 pints) of water per day, either as pure water or herbal teas. If your urine is darker than a pale straw colour, then it's a sign you need to drink more water!

What to limit in your diet during perimenopause

Now I know no-one wants a list of food they can't eat, but there are some foods that can worsen perimenopause symptoms and increase the risk of long-term health conditions. Limiting these can go a long way in supporting your well-being now and in the future:

Sugar & High GL Carbs: Sugar and foods like white bread, pasta, rice, potatoes and baked goods, can lead to blood sugar spikes, cravings and weight gain.

Processed Foods: One of the most important shifts you can make in perimenopause is stepping away from convenience and processed foods. Packed full of refined sugars, unhealthy fats, artificial additives and preservatives, these foods can wreak havoc on our health and hormones.

Caffeine: Although coffee may have health benefits, many women don't tolerate caffeine well during perimenopause and it can worsen anxiety, hot flashes, and sleep disturbances. Consider transitioning to herbal teas or stick to just 1-2 cups of good quality coffee earlier in the day.

Alcohol: Alcohol may provide momentary pleasure, but it can exacerbate symptoms like hot flashes, night sweats, mood swings, sleep issues, anxiety, and depression. The best advice is to avoid alcohol altogether, but if this is a step too far for you, try cutting back a bit and see if your symptoms improve.

Spicy foods: If you're experiencing hot flashes and night sweats, you may want to cut back on spicy foods as these can bring your body temperature up, triggering or exacerbating symptoms.

In conclusion

Remember there is no one-size-fits-all diet in perimenopause – we are all unique and our bodies have different needs. However, focusing on wholesome, nourishing foods and following these general guidelines, can make a huge difference to your well-being and your experience of perimenopause. I encourage you to really embrace this time to take charge of your health and use the power of nutrition to support you now and in the future. Your body and mind will thank you for it.

Helen x

If you would like to know more about how nutritional therapy can improve your well-being during perimenopause and beyond, you can book a free, no-obligation call with me:

Notes:

CHAPTER ELEVEN
Embracing Change:
5 Steps to Cultivate a
Positive Mindset During
Perimenopause
by Debi Haden

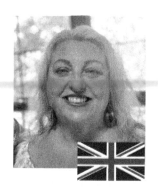

Bio: Debi is a Mindset and Mindfulness Coach. Maintaining a positive mindset can lead to positive life outcomes, even when navigating significant life changes such as perimenopause and menopause. Each woman's situation is unique, and my approach is tailored accordingly. I aim to provide you with a comprehensive support package, empowering you to regain strength and control your life.

Business: Debi Haden - Dare to Shine
Website: www.debihaden.com

Perimenopause, often referred to as the "change before the change," is a unique and transformative phase in a woman's life. It's a time when the body undergoes profound hormonal shifts, leading to a range of physical and emotional changes. These changes can be challenging, but they also offer an opportunity for growth, self-discovery, and a renewed sense of purpose.

In this chapter, we will explore five essential steps to help you cultivate a positive mindset during perimenopause. These steps are not just about managing symptoms; they're about embracing this transition with grace and resilience, empowering yourself with knowledge, and discovering the beauty that can come with change.

Step 1: Self-Compassion - Nurturing Yourself Through Change

Perimenopause is often accompanied by a myriad of physical symptoms and emotional fluctuations. It's easy to be critical of yourself during this time, but self-compassion is the foundation upon which a positive mindset is built.

Understanding Self-Compassion

Self-compassion is the practice of treating yourself with the same kindness, love, and understanding that you would offer to a dear friend. It involves acknowledging your challenges, accepting your imperfections, and embracing your vulnerability. Here's how to nurture self-compassion:

Practice Self-Talk: Pay attention to your inner dialogue. When you catch yourself being overly critical or judgmental, pause and reframe your thoughts with self-compassion. Instead of saying, "I can't believe I'm so moody," try saying, "I'm navigating a challenging phase, and it's okay to have ups and downs."

Self-Care Rituals: Prioritise self-care activities that make you feel nurtured and grounded. This could include indulging in a warm bath, practising gentle yoga, or simply enjoying a quiet moment with a cup of tea.

Mindful Self-Awareness: Develop mindful awareness of your emotions and body. When you experience discomfort or frustration, acknowledge it without judgement. Say to yourself, "This is a difficult moment, and it's okay to feel this way."

Seek Support: Lean on your support network, whether it's your partner, friends, or a support group. Sharing your experiences and feelings with others who understand can provide comfort and a sense of community.

Set Realistic Expectations: Understand that perimenopause can be challenging, but it doesn't mean you have to be perfect. Set realistic expectations for yourself, and don't be too hard on yourself when things don't go as planned.

Self-compassion is not about indulging in self-pity, but about treating yourself with kindness and understanding. It's the first step toward embracing change with an open heart.

Step 2: Knowledge is Empowerment – Understanding Perimenopause

Knowledge is a powerful tool when it comes to navigating perimenopause. Understanding the science behind perimenopause, its symptoms, and the changes happening in your body empowers you to make informed decisions about your health and well-being.

Harnessing the Power of Knowledge

- **Seek Reliable Sources:** Begin your journey by seeking information from reputable sources, such as healthcare professionals, books, and trusted websites dedicated to women's health. Avoid relying solely on anecdotal stories or unverified advice.

- **Consult Your Healthcare Provider:** Your healthcare provider is a valuable resource during perimenopause. They can provide tailored guidance, discuss treatment options, and address your specific concerns. Don't hesitate to ask questions and seek clarification about any aspect of perimenopause.

- **Track Your Symptoms:** Keep a journal or use a dedicated app to track your symptoms. This can help you identify patterns, triggers, and changes over time, providing valuable insights for both you and your healthcare provider.

- **Join Supportive Communities:** Consider joining support groups or online forums where women going through perimenopause share their experiences. These communities can provide emotional support and valuable insights from those who understand what you're going through.

- **Stay Updated:** Perimenopause research is ongoing, and new insights emerge regularly. Stay updated with the latest findings to ensure your knowledge remains current and accurate.

Understanding the science behind perimenopause and being informed about your options for symptom management gives you the tools to make choices that align with your needs and preferences.

Step 3: Mindfulness and Meditation – Cultivating Inner Peace

The emotional rollercoaster of perimenopause can be intense, but mindfulness and meditation can be powerful tools to help you stay present in the moment, manage stress, and nurture your emotional well-being.

Embracing Mindfulness and Meditation

Mindful Awareness: Practice mindfulness by consciously observing your thoughts, emotions, and bodily sensations without judgement. This awareness helps you detach from the automatic reactions triggered by emotional fluctuations.

Deep Breathing: Engage in deep breathing exercises to calm your nervous system. Simply taking a few moments to focus on your breath can help alleviate stress and anxiety.

Mindful Eating: Apply mindfulness to your eating habits.

Pay attention to the flavours, textures, and sensations of your food. This practice can enhance your relationship with food and promote healthier choices.

Meditation Sessions: Set aside time for meditation sessions, even if they're just a few minutes each day. Guided meditations, meditation apps, or classes can provide structure and guidance if you're new to meditation.

Yoga Practice: Consider incorporating yoga into your routine. Yoga combines physical postures, breath control, and mindfulness, offering a holistic approach to physical and emotional well-being.

Mindfulness and meditation promote a sense of inner calm, resilience, and self-awareness. They can help you navigate the ups and downs of perimenopause with greater ease and grace.

Step 4: Support Network – Building a Circle of Understanding

A support network is a crucial element in your journey through perimenopause. Your loved ones, friends, or a support group can provide emotional support, understanding, and a sense of community during this transformative phase.

Leveraging Your Support Network

Open Communication: Share your experiences and feelings with your support network. Let them know what you're going through and how they can best support you. Open and honest communication is key to building a strong support system.

Lean on Loved Ones: Your partner, if you have one, can be an incredible source of support. Talk to them about your needs, and involve them in your journey. Their understanding and empathy can make a significant difference.

Friends and Family: Don't hesitate to reach out to close friends and family members. They may not fully grasp what perimenopause entails, but they can still offer a listening ear and emotional support.

Support Groups: Consider joining a local or online support group specifically focused on perimenopause or menopause. These groups provide a safe space to share experiences, ask questions, and receive support from individuals who understand the unique challenges of this phase.

Professional Help: If you're struggling with severe emotional symptoms or mental health issues during perimenopause, seeking the assistance of a therapist or counsellor can be immensely beneficial.

Remember that you don't have to navigate perimenopause alone. Building a strong support network can provide a sense of belonging and emotional security, which is vital for maintaining a positive mindset.

Step 5: Adapt and Embrace – Thriving Amidst Change

The final step in cultivating a positive mindset during perimenopause is to adapt to the changes happening in your body and embrace the opportunities this phase offers.

Embracing Adaptation

Flexibility: Embrace flexibility in your daily routines and expectations. Understand that your energy levels, moods, and physical comfort may vary from day to day. Be willing to adjust your plans accordingly.

Discover New Passions: Use this phase as an opportunity to discover new passions and interests. Explore hobbies or activities that you've always wanted to try. Engaging in activities you enjoy can boost your mood and self-esteem.

Prioritise Self-Care: Make self-care a non-negotiable part of your routine. This includes getting adequate rest, eating nourishing foods, engaging in regular physical activity, and managing stress through relaxation techniques.

Embrace Change: Instead of resisting change, view it as a chance for personal growth and renewal. Perimenopause is a transitional phase, and by embracing the changes, you can emerge from it stronger and more resilient.

Set Goals: Continue setting goals and aspirations for

yourself. Whether they're related to your career, personal development, or relationships, having goals can provide a sense of purpose and direction.

Adapting to the changes of perimenopause and embracing new opportunities can lead to a more positive outlook on life. It's a reminder that this phase, like all others, is part of your unique journey, and it's filled with possibilities.

Cultivating a positive mindset during perimenopause is not a linear journey. It involves self-compassion, knowledge, mindfulness, a support network, and a willingness to adapt. By embracing these five steps, you can navigate the challenges of perimenopause with grace, resilience, and a sense of empowerment.

Remember that you are not alone on this journey, and with the right mindset, you can embrace change and emerge from perimenopause as a stronger and wiser version of yourself.

You've got this!

You are welcome to contact me on debi@debihaden.com for a FREE 30-minute conversation about how I can help and support you as you go through this next stage of your journey.

After reading this chapter...

What one action can you take immediately?

What one action can you take next week?

What one action can you take a month from now?

What are you telling yourself about going through this stage of your life?

What do you want to tell yourself instead?

What do you need to do to allow yourself to *shine* again?

"A strong woman knows she has strength enough for the journey,
but a woman of strength knows it is in the journey where she will
become strong."

CHAPTER TWELVE
The Missing Piece in Your Perimenopause Exercise Puzzle (it's not what you think)
by Tracy Seider

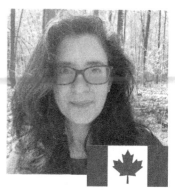

Bio: Tracy Seider is a corrective exercise specialist for peri/menopausal women who are DONE with their stiff, achy, stuck-behind-screens bodies and are ready to get in shape, feel ache-free, and age well - WITHOUT the sweat, strain, or time-suck of traditional exercise.

Tracy's simpler, smarter, science-based Reshape Method™ program gives women the confidence, strength & energy to show up every day, ready to CRUSH their life & work goals ... NOW - and well into the future.

Business Name: Tracy Seider Coaching
Website: https://tracyseidercoaching.com/

"At 53, I'm stronger, slimmer, ache-free and happier than I was 10 years ago.
Am I special? NO.
Do I have a special approach ? Heck, YES!"

[WARNING: Barbie dolls were harmed in the writing of this chapter.]

As a Peri/menopause Corrective Exercise Specialist and founding expert in the Perimenopause Hub Facebook community, I'm tickled pink to be included in this volume alongside other outstanding health and wellness professionals, who are united in our common mission to help perimenopausal women to not just survive this challenging change, but to (in the words of Hub founder, Emily Barclay) feel EPIC.

And *EXERCISE* is an important part of this.

In fact, when it comes to looking great, feeling great, and thriving through the menopause transition, exercise ranks right up there with good nutrition, proper sleep, and hormone therapy (where appropriate), and is specifically recommended by leading menopause experts such as Dr Jen Gunter[1] and Dr Louann Brizendine.[2]

This probably comes as no surprise. After all, we've been told since we were kids that exercise is good for us. But declining estrogen levels, and the subsequent loss of its protective effects through perimenopause and beyond, takes the importance of regular exercise to a whole new level. That's because exercise has been shown to provide key benefits when it comes to specific areas that affect peri/menopausal women, such as

---

[1] Gunter, J. The Menopause Manifesto: Own Your Health With Facts and Feminimism. Toronto: Random House Canada, 2021
[2] Brizendine, L. The Upgrade: How the Female Brain Gets Stronger and Better in Midlife and Beyond. New York: Harmony Books, 2022.

weight management, type 2 diabetes, hot flashes, mood and stress management, brain health, bone health, heart health, and more.

Some specific exercise recommendations for perimenopausal women include:

Daily **walking.**

Weaving 10,000 steps into your day is a great way to get natural movement and to break up our often sedentary lifestyle - especially if your work has you stuck behind screens. Plus, the sunlight exposure is important for mood, Vitamin D production, and maintaining a good circadian rhythm, which helps with sleep.

Some **cardio** or high-intensity interval training (HIIT).

Not too much though because, at perimenopause, spikes in cortisol levels caused by intense exercise can actually contribute to belly fat, muscle loss, and insomnia.

Some **stretching, mindfulness and core strengthening** exercise, like yoga or Pilates.

And last but not least, **strength training** or resistance workouts that build muscle.

Building muscle should be a priority at perimenopause. This is because muscle mass peaks in our 20s and declines from then on due to age and dropping estrogen levels. And muscle is a menopausal secret weapon: it gets your metabolism going and gives you a great shape; it's a key part of osteoporosis prevention and treatment; and building muscle in the right areas can resolve many aches and pains. Plus, muscle is what helps you to age well – keeping you agile, anti-frail, and independent.

So, following these recommendations to move more, many perimenopausal women take up exercise, or commit to new or more exercise as part of a midlife wellness protocol. Except, despite good intentions, when it comes to exercise, things are often not plain sailing – and it's common to see posts like this in the Perimenopause Hub Facebook group.

"Looking for suggestions and support. I'm 45 and feeling pretty miserable. I have nagging hip, back and foot pain. I spend my life at physical therapy, chiropractor and massage appointments. I feel better for a day or two, but then the aches come right back. I can't focus on my work and dread the thought of having to sit at my computer, knowing how sore I'll be at the end of the day.

I've been for loads of tests. The doctor says I'm fine – I just need to exercise more and take pain meds as needed. But the more I exercise (treadmill, elliptical, bike) the worse my hip pain. Walking isn't an option because of the foot pain, plus my back aches if I walk too far. I'm forever putting my neck out, and my shoulders are so tight, even though I do yoga regularly and teach a few classes a week.

I've tried orthotics, different mattresses, countless office chairs – nothing makes a difference.

The hip pain keeps me up at night, as do the trips to the bathroom. I'm so tired, and I snap at my husband and daughters. I hate who I've become.

Also, my shape has changed, and the weight won't budge no matter how much I exercise.

I feel like I've lost control of my body and don't recognize myself anymore – that it really is all downhill from here.

But I'm too young to feel so old. I was not expecting this."

Now, don't worry, I haven't broken any Facebook group privacy rules by sharing this quote.

You see, this was MY reality eight years ago – and if the Perimenopause Hub had been around in 2015, that is likely what I would have posted. But, back then, I hadn't even heard of the term 'perimenopause', and it would be another four years until the Hub was established. So I struggled alone, getting increasingly dejected and frustrated because I was not seeing results for the amount of time and effort I was putting into exercise.

Also, instead of helping me to feel better, exercise was making me feel WORSE. It was exacerbating my existing aches and pains, and causing new injuries (like the lower back injury I got when I started weight training), which meant I had to cut back or quit exercising until I felt better.

And, as I'm sure you've experienced, it's really hard to return to exercise after a setback, especially when as a working, 'sandwich' generation perimenopausal woman, finding the time, energy, and motivation to exercise is a struggle to start with. However, a part of me believed that these issues were NOT just a normal part of aging - as I was being told.

I was sure I was missing something ... but had no idea what that something could be as I was already doing all the 'right' things. But I kept searching and researching, and my tenacity eventually paid off - because, at 53, I'm stronger, slimmer, ache-free and happier than I was 10 years ago. I sleep like a baby, and no longer dress strategically to hide the lumps and bumps. I exercise LESS and eat MORE. My plantar fasciitis is gone, and so are my orthotics.

And while I'm still stuck behind screens, teaching my online Reshape Method™ corrective exercise program to hundreds of women around the world, my hip and back pain are a thing of the past, and I'm having a mostly symptom-free perimenopause.

Am I special?

NO.

Do I know the missing piece in the perimenopause exercise puzzle?

Heck, YES!

You're in for a surprise, though, because that elusive missing piece is not more exercise, or trying the latest workout craze, or even finding the right personal trainer or yoga teacher.

It's **ALIGNMENT**.

Yep, the missing piece in the perimenopause exercise puzzle is less about WHAT exercise you do, how much of it you get, or what heart rate you reach, and more about HOW your body is able to do a particular exercise or movement, based on your body's alignment.

You see, as moving, mechanical animals there is a default, factory specification setting from which the human body can best move. This default position allows for maximum force generation from our muscles (so you get more bang for your exercise buck), and ensures minimal wear and tear and inflammation on our joints (no aches, injuries, or setbacks).

That magical position is called anatomical neutral - like the skeleton back in your high school biology classroom ... or like my daughter's new Barbie doll.

(Granted, Barbie's proportions aren't realistic, but she works for general illustration purposes.)

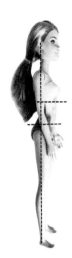 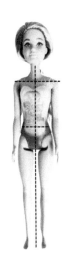

You see, Neutral Barbie represents optimal alignment because, from the side, I can draw a straight line through the centre of her ear, shoulder, hip, knee, and ankle. Her pelvis is not tipped forward or titled backwards, and her neutral ribcage rests directly above her neutral pelvis.

From the front, when I draw a straight line through the middle of Neutral Barbie's body, her hips are even and so are her shoulders.

(This Barbie's heels touch the ground, where they belong, else she wouldn't be in anatomical neutral. And neither are you, for that matter, if your shoes have you in a heel - however slight the lift.)

A body that generally comes to rest in an anatomically neutral position is what we should be aiming for because, in anatomical neutral, our bones are at specific angles relative to each other and relative to gravity so that minimal stress is applied to our muscles, tendons, nerves and bones when we move, and so that we can get the most stability, balance, strength, and power from that movement.

The thing is, once I learned about alignment, I realized that while I had good 'posture' …

(I habitually forced a chest up, shoulders back, belly in posture that was drilled into me as a kid, thinking it was the 'right' thing to do - it's not!) … the shape of my body from a biomechanical perspective did not resemble Neutral Barbie's.

On closer inspection, I looked more like Miss Aligned Barbie 1.

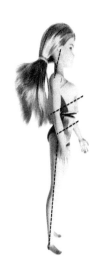

- My leg was not fully vertical to the ground, but actually diagonal
- My pelvis was tipped forward and hiked up to the right
- My rib cage was lifted, thrust forward, and twisted to the right
- My shoulders, when I was not forcing them back, were hunched and sitting up by my ears (not shown on this Barbie; the model has its limitations, but you get the gist)
- And I had Forward Head Posture and the beginnings of a neck hump!

This meant that the body I was exercising (or even just

walking around the block) could not move as designed.

Instead, my movements were created from a series of 'cheats' and compensatory patterns, which, in my 40s, were now catching up with me.

So while I was moving ... I could not move well, even if I tried.

But, as Dr Phil says, you can't change what you don't acknowledge.

And everything did change when I finally understood that the REAL root cause of my issues was that I was misaligned. Not that I wasn't active enough, or strong enough, or supple enough, or too old, or not trying hard enough. My issues were not even perimenopause related, but more the fact that the hormonal changes of perimenopause tend to happen at an age when our bodies can no longer mask or manage these misalignments and accompanying movement cheats.

(Misalignments often mean we're over-using certain muscles that shouldn't be moving us, and under-using muscles that SHOULD be moving us.)

But when I gave myself the grace and space STOP 'exercising' and instead took a back-to-basics approach, reshaping my body into better alignment through the right mix of dynamic corrective exercises, functional movement, and habit changes - that's when the magic really started to happen.

You see, I needed to slow down in order to speed up.

So, if exercise is not giving you the shape and pain-free living results you want, it may be because you are also out of alignment from years of modern living. Your misalignments may resemble mine, or they may look more like Miss Aligned Barbie 2 (tucked pelvis, ribcage pulled down), or you may be a combination of these and more, because misalignments are as individual as the person.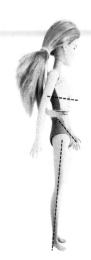

Either way, the thing to remember is that when you are misaligned, your body can no longer move as designed. This means that exercising more, or harder, will likely just give you the same results. So, to get more bang for your exercise buck at perimenopause (and to stop getting injured trying) taking a step back, hitting the reset button, and reshaping your body from the inside out FIRST, may be what's missing for you too.

Take this Posture and Alignment Quiz to see if alignment is the missing piece in YOUR perimenopause exercise puzzle.

Journal Prompt:

Next steps I want to take…

"The definition of 'insanity' is doing the same thing over and over again and expecting different results." – Albert Einstein

CHAPTER THIRTEEN
From Farm to Fork: The Impact of Food Production on our Hormones
by Ruby Saharan, B.Sc., M.Sc., INHC.

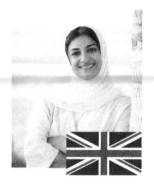

Bio: Hi there! I'm Ruby, an Integrative Nutrition Practitioner, with over 15 years of experience working in the Healthcare Industry. I help professional women overcome Hormonal Imbalance by improving their digestive health using The Hormone Reset Roadmap©- a simple program that doesn't involve strict diets or difficult exercise regimes. I've written this chapter to help women like you make informed choices when choosing what to eat. I hope you find it useful!

Business: Jigsaw Wellness Ltd.
Website: www.jigsaw-wellness.com

This chapter is all about modern agriculture and how raising animals and growing produce can affect women's hormonal health. Find out:

· *How industrial farming has changed our environment.*
· *Why this can impact your hormones.*
· *Ways to "clean up" your diet and what to look out for.*

Modern agriculture has transformed the way we produce food, enabling the world to sustain a growing population. The food industry has grown exponentially over the last century and continues to usher in foods based on convenience and accessibility. However, with the advent of industrialised farming practices, concerns have been raised about the potential impact on human health- including hormonal disruption.

Farming practices significantly impact gut health and consequently, hormone health. Things like pesticides and synthetic fertilisers can leave residual chemicals in our food, potentially disrupting the delicate environment of the gut. These disruptions in the gut microbiome have been linked to hormonal imbalance in women which can make the journey of perimenopause rockier than it should be! Don't worry though - I'll reveal what you can do about it in this chapter, so read on to the end!

Before we begin: Please note that the information in this chapter is not medical advice- if you're inspired after reading this, consult a qualified healthcare practitioner before making any drastic changes to what you eat.

Raising Animals & Hormone Disruption

"The Health of The Animal Affects the Health of The Consumer!"

Headlines have scared us off eating meat products for decades, but are they true? I know I've grown up feeling conflicted and confused at times. Concerns dramatically highlighted by the media surround the manufacturing and consumption of animal products; including use of antibiotics, factory farming, animal cruelty, cloning, irradiation, toxic sludge, E. coli bacteria, mad cow disease, hormone administration, genetic engineering, bovine growth hormone, cancer, heart disease, obesity, constipation... the list goes on!

What's going on? Are we all going to get sick? Is the modern perimenopausal woman doomed? Let's look at the facts:

In industrialised farming, the use of synthetic hormones to enhance livestock growth and increase milk production is widespread. Hormones such as oestrogen, progesterone, and testosterone can be administered to livestock to promote growth, increase milk production, or improve reproductive efficiency.

There is also established evidence indicating that hormones from livestock can enter the human body through consumption of meat and dairy products [1], [2].

Whilst the levels of hormones found in these products are generally considered to be low and unlikely to cause significant hormonal disruptions, it is recognized that *some* transfer of hormones can occur. The same goes for antibiotics.

[1] Schdrader & Cooke, (2000) Exposure of the U.S. Population to Estrogens; Journal of Environmental Health Perspectives. 2000 Jun;108(Suppl 4):791-3. Link: https://pubmed.ncbi.nlm.nih.gov/10852853/
[2] Sharpe RR, Smith BB, Coeling Mercer MS. (1991) The Transfer of 17β-Estradiol to Dairy Milk in Cows; J Dairy Sci. 1991 Dec;74(12):4238-43. Link: https://pubmed.ncbi.nlm.nih.gov/1818223/

So, on one hand we have evidence suggesting that hormone and antibiotic residues from treated animals may be found in animal products, and on the other a consensus in the scientific community that the levels in meat and dairy from treated animals is low enough to be safe.

Other factors to consider are the environment and feed of the animal. Grass-fed livestock is free to roam, and its produce has a better nutritional profile. Grain-fed livestock on the other hand, is given a diet of (mostly) GM corn and soy. This results in meat and dairy that is of lower quality and higher in fatty acids that cause increased cholesterol in humans.

With all this said, you may now be wondering whether it's good to avoid animal products, and I don't blame you! It can be a bit of a minefield. How much and what types of protein one should consume is highly debated and people can be very passionate about their protein choice.

Some say high-quality animal protein is needed for optimal health, whilst others advocate for a plant-based diet. I would say arm yourself with knowledge and experiment with what works for your body at this time in your life. That way you'll be able to successfully guide yourself to your appropriate protein source. Under the guidance of a nutrition specialist this approach can be very powerful for improving Hormonal Health. Be aware that peri-and post-menopausal women need more protein than younger women. Healthy protein intake is essential to prevent complications later in life such as osteoarthritis and muscle loss.

It is also worth knowing that we do need to consume whole proteins (as well as healthy fats) to produce good quality hormones in our bodies. It is trickier (not impossible!) to get the full range of amino acids our bodies need from a vegetarian or vegan diet, so consult a nutrition professional if you don't eat any meat and/or dairy to check you are getting everything you need.

If you do choose to eat animal proteins, I always advise to eat high-quality, organic, free-range, grass-fed forms. The health of the animal affects the health of the consumer!

Pesticides

"Nobody Knows What Level of Exposure is Safe for Long-Term Hormone Health"

In large-scale industrial farming, fields grow one type of crop year after year and are treated with pesticides, herbicides, and synthetic fertilisers. It has allowed us to increase crop yields and keep up with growing populations. However, these chemicals can seep into the soil and water, contaminating food sources and impacting hormonal health.

Let's delve in... What's the actual scientific evidence out there? Is this more scaremongering? Or do we all need to start growing our own veg and living on farms?

The use of pesticides in modern agriculture has raised concerns about impact on hormonal health for years. Many pesticides have been linked to endocrine disruption. A recent scientific review of the latest evidence found that environmental exposure to hormone disrupting chemicals could even contribute to earlier menopause [3]. Another review published in The Lancet by Kahn et.al., (2020)[4] reported associations between pesticide exposure and lower progesterone levels, and an increased risk of irregular menstrual cycles in women. There are many more studies- both in animals and humans that demonstrate a clear link between pesticide exposure and hormonal disruption.

Governments and regulators try their best to keep us all safe, whilst ensuring everyone has enough to eat- but the reality is that nobody knows what level of exposure is safe for long-term hormone health. There are little to no robust studies looking at this in perimenopausal women.

From the information available, I think we can safely conclude that over-exposure to commercial pesticides is not going to be good for any of us!

So, what do we do? Well, what we know for sure is that around 63% of commercial produce will retain one or more traces of pesticide- even after washing. A good starting point is to look up the official "Dirty Dozen" list for your country. This identifies commercial produce most contaminated with residues from pesticides and you can use it to guide your weekly shopping choices. It is published by non-profit

[3]Neff, A., Laws, M., Warner, G., & Flaws, J. (2022). The Effects of Environmental Contaminant Exposure on Reproductive Aging and the Menopause Transition. Current Environmental Health Reports, 9(1), 53-79.
[4] Kahn et al, 2020 Endocrine-disrupting chemicals: implications for human health The Lancet endocrine-disrupting chemicals| volume 8, issue 8, p703-718, August 2020 DOI:https://doi.org/10.1016/S2213-8587(20)30129-7

organisations, namely the Environmental Working group (www.ewg.org) in the USA and the Pesticide Action Network (www.pan-uk.org) in the UK.

It's a simple way to reduce exposure to toxic synthetic pesticides used on fruits and vegetables. Another alternative is to buy organic. I always advise clients to consider organic farms for produce and buy local where possible. Being realistic, you won't ever dodge every single pesticide (unless you literally do have your own self-sustained farm!) but the idea is to lower your personal exposure as much as possible.

Genetically Modified Organisms (GMOs)

"80% of Processed Food and most Fast Foods contain some GMOs"

GMOs are plants or animals that have had their DNA modified. They are plants or animals that have been genetically engineered with DNA from bacteria, viruses, or other plants and animals.

GM crops were first introduced in the USA in 1994 with the Flavr Savr tomato, which had been genetically modified to slow its ripening process, delaying softening and rotting. The farming of GM crops has massively increased since then.

In 2015, GM crops were grown in 28 countries and on 179.7 million hectares – that is over 10% of the world's arable land. Most corn, soybean, cotton, and canola crops are now genetically modified.

In fact, in 2015, 83% of the world's production of soybean, 75% of cotton, 29% of maize and 25% of rapeseed oil production was genetically modified (www.royalsociety.org). The USA, Brazil and Argentina are the leading producers. There are currently no GM crops being grown commercially in the UK although scientists are carrying out controlled trials.

What you need to know is that many of these crops are then used in processed foodstuffs including cooking oils, specialist starch (often added to foods like coatings and batters) and other food ingredients. For example, processed foods, cooking oil, sauces, biscuits, and confectionery made from or containing GM crops – which must be labelled as such – are available in UK supermarkets. The hard fact is that *nearly 80% of processed food and most fast food contain GMOs.*

So, what does this mean for our hormones? Well, as before, sadly the data is lacking. There is no evidence for or against GMOs and our perimenopausal hormone health. That said, evidence is mounting that genetically modified food crops may be a cause of infertility, so we do know that they are affecting our hormones somehow!

The easiest and best thing we can do is to avoid processed foods that contain corn syrup, high fructose corn syrup, processed sugar, fillers, soybean oil, cottonseed oil, canola oil, rapeseed oil, artificial flavours or colours. Read labels carefully and stick to foods as close to their natural state as possible-your hormones will thank you!

To conclude, modern agriculture has undoubtedly helped us to produce food on a large scale, but it comes with significant consequences for our hormonal health. It's high time we all thought about preserving and co-existing with the environment whilst eating better.

Transitioning towards organic and sustainable food sources is crucial for both our well-being and the future of farming. Embracing organic foods not only nurtures our health but also fosters a healthier ecosystem. By reducing our reliance on synthetic chemicals and GMOs, we will promote cleaner soil, water, air, human and animal health. Replacing industrial meat and dairy with organic, grass-fed options will ensure that livestock are raised in humane conditions, translating into better quality products for consumers. It's better for all of us, and is certainly "food for thought".

Sounds great on paper right? But what about the reality? The reality is, we're a bunch of stressed-out women with a lot on our midlife minds. We are dealing with the physical changes, often have teens to deal with along with other family relationships and careers to maintain. The reality is we reach out for familiar foods more often than we like, and it is difficult to break down habits of a lifetime. We need to eat quick- and sometimes just don't have the bandwidth to think about our own health or figure out whether we are eating the right quantities of the right stuff.

Sound familiar? Would you like help with the mental load of creating sustainable diet & lifestyle shifts?

I am offering a complimentary NutriScan©, exclusive only to readers of this book. During your NutriScan©, I will assess your current diet and give you a FREE 3-Point Action Plan to implement straight away, tailored to YOU.

To book yours, just click on the QR code and mention that you are a reader.

It's all completely free and there are no obligations at all. Give it a go- you never know, this might be the beginning of an exciting health transformation- just like it has been for my clients!

Notes:

I will swap out these foods for better options on my next food shopping trip:

"Eating Knowledgeably is the Absolute Foundation for a Healthy Journey to Menopause and Beyond"

CHAPTER FOURTEEN
Ditch the Fawn, Embrace
the Fierce
by Kirsten Alberts

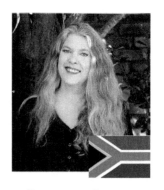

Bio: I am a Support and Trauma Counsellor specialising in identifying and breaking toxic patterns.

Business: Kirsten Alberts Counselling
Website: www.kirstenalberts.co.za

Do you find yourself: "Rescuing" everybody all the time? Being everyone's support but your own? Having trouble setting boundaries, or saying "NO"?

Most people have heard of "Fight" or "Flight" when responding to stressful or dangerous situations. But have you heard of "Fawn"?

Do you find yourself "rescuing" everybody all the time? Being everyone's support system but your own? Having trouble standing up for yourself, setting boundaries, and saying "no"? Repeatedly forgiving people who refuse to change? Hyper-sensitive to people's moods? Feeling the need to be "useful" all the time? Then "fawn" is probably your stress response.

Fawning is learned (or more sinisterly, encouraged) in childhood as a way to face physical and emotionally threatening situations. It's the way we "please and appease" our way out of harm's way. We learn that if we are nice, or helpful, or obedient, then we have a better chance at minimising the threat, and surviving another day. While fawning may have served us in childhood when we had no other choice but to please and placate the people who hurt us, fawning does NOT serve us as adults. All it does is cement that we "shouldn't make a fuss" or "cause an upset", and before we know it, we are people-pleasing doormats, wondering how the hell we got here, and why we are so unhappy about it.

Here are six ways to ditch the Fawn, and embrace the Fierce. But, it comes with a warning label: Some people are NOT going to like this AT ALL. Why would they? They have enjoyed the perks and benefits of exploiting your lovely nature for years. Now you want it all to change? How very dare you. These are the people who are going to say: "What's gotten into to her?", "She's falling off the rails", "Going bonkers". Don't fall for it. Simply put, those who don't like your boundaries, benefit from you not having any in the first place. The upside is, you will soon see that there is a different set of people altogether. Those who will love your anti-doormat process, and applaud you for it. These are your people. And the more time you spend with people who admire and support you, the faster you will learn to stop worrying about what everybody else thinks, and start living a life that doesn't centre around what you can do for them.

1. Ask yourself how you genuinely feel versus how pressured you feel.

When someone asks you to do something, instead of automatically jumping to say "yes", pause, take a breath, and ask yourself if you really WANT to say yes. Do you have the time? The energy? The money? Is it something this person can do for themselves? Will you have to reorganise your plans, go out of your way, or skip something you have already arranged? Maybe it's something you disagree with, feel uncomfortable doing, or simply don't want to be doing. Perhaps it is something that you keep doing, so this person never learns to do it for themselves. Figure out whether you are giving in to the pressure of saying yes versus actually wanting to.

2. Separate the perceived benefits from actual consequences.

When we are children, there are some benefits to fawning. Placating our tormentors meant evading a physical blow or a psychological attack. The more it worked, the more we fawned, so the more we believed that it was a perfectly good strategy to keep ourselves safe. What we don't realise as adults, is that fawning only kept us safe, as children, in that moment. It did nothing to teach us boundaries, or how to say no, because the consequences of standing up for ourselves would have been terrifying. The consequences of fawning as adults are completely different. We may benefit from people-pleasing by feeling good and safe in the moment, but it's more likely to get us walked all over, taken advantage of, and outright exploited in the long run. Most people tend to treat others according to what they tolerate, so if you are tolerating disrespect, manipulation and exploitation, you will be expected to keep tolerating it, and like it. Make a list of the pros and cons of immediate benefits versus long-term consequences. It will help you to see that fawning isn't beneficial at all.

3. Get angry.

Ask yourself how fairly you are being treated. Do people make demands on you that they would never dream of making on anyone else? If you are unable to jump to those demands, are you punished in any way? Are you subject to sulking? Rage? Or the silent treatment? Do you deserve to be? Then ask yourself how these events SHOULD have played out. How SHOULD these people have behaved, and how SHOULD you have been treated?

4. What would you tell a friend?

If a friend was being exploited and asked you for advice, what would you tell them? Would you express dismay at how unfairly they are being treated? Would you agree that their feelings are valid? Offer boundary ideas? Even suggest ways they could escape the situation entirely? Fawning is often accompanied by a history of negative self-talk copied from how we were spoken to as children. If we hear that we are "lazy, stupid, selfish" often enough, especially by the people we have no option but to trust, we really have no option but to believe it. So we learn that if we are our own harshest critics, we can avoid making any mistakes that will earn us a beating or berating. If we treat ourselves the way we would a beloved friend, we start to see just how awful our inner critic can be, who put the critic there in the first place, and just how badly we've been beating ourselves up for mistakes we didn't make.

5. Stop kneecapping yourself.

"Kneecapping" is the act of incapacitating someone by shooting them in the knee. When we use modifiers such as: "just", "maybe" and "sort of", we think we are softening our words, but all we're doing is incapacitating ourselves. "That sort of makes me feel uncomfortable." "Maybe you should leave." "I just want to remind you that this project is due tomorrow." Take those kneecapping words out, and reread each sentence. See what I mean?

6. Learn that "no" isn't a dirty word.

Or if you're like me and you like dirty words, this one is extra special. It is also a complete sentence. If you're just getting started, try: "Thanks, but I already have plans" in response to a texted invitation. Don't be tempted to add page-long explanations as to what those plans are and why you can't make it to your sister-in-law's super-fun tupperware party. (You could be pyjama-binge-watching Netflix. Plans are plans). Your time is your own to use as you see fit, and only you know how much time your family, career, and goals need to keep them running healthily. Please don't spend time on explaining how you spend time. That is way too much spending, and not enough binging.

Power through your urge to J.A.D.E: Justify, Argue, Defend, Explain. There are very few people who deserve an explanation as to what you are doing with your time. Your bitchy sister-in-law isn't one of them.

Email me at: info@kirstenalberts.co.za

Journal Prompts:

What kinds of favours do I feel pressured into doing? By whom?

What are the short-term effects of my fawning, and how do I think my fawning will affect me in the future?

What makes me angry after I have fawned?

What advice would I give to an unhappy friend who fawned instead of saying "No"?

Which kneecapping words do I use?

Did I say "No" today?

Your Story Matters.

CHAPTER FIFTEEN
Ease Your Symptoms
with Food As Medicine
by Laura Viale

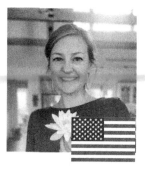

Bio: Laura is a Functional Nutrition Counselor and an Ayurvedic Lifestyle Coach specializing in hormone balance for women in peri and post-menopause. She is the founder of Naturally Thriving Women's Health, and she is passionate about teaching women how to use the science of Functional Nutrition and the wisdom of Ayurveda to honor their bodies, trust in their own wisdom, and Thrive through the stages of menopause and beyond.

Business: Naturally Thriving Women's Health
Website: www.naturallythriving.health

Food has the power to make your symptoms go away, or make them WAY worse

Learn how the science of Functional Nutrition, paired with the wisdom of Ayurveda can make your symptoms fade away, boost your energy, boost your mood and help you feel like yourself again. Healing and balancing your mind and body from the inside out allows you to trust, love and appreciate your incredible body.

The POWER of Food:

What I've found through personal experience and after helping hundreds of women get their energy back, sleep better, maintain a healthy weight and feel more alive - is that food has the power to make your symptoms go away, or make them WAY worse.

The concept of using food as medicine dates back centuries, as various cultures have recognized the powerful impact of nutrient-rich diets on overall health. But what excites me - even after spending over 20 years helping my clients step into their healthiest lives - is how deeply and quickly food can make an impact on specific areas of health. This absolutely includes hormone health and easing the symptoms associated with the stages of menopause.

We know that key nutrients and compounds found in high quality veggies, fruits, whole grains, animal and plant proteins, and healthy fats can make a profound impact on our hormone health. Similarly, we can choose to minimize eating foods that are known hormone disruptors like refined sugar, dairy, and gluten.

When our body's key systems are functioning well, and when we understand how to balance our meals in the right combination for our body type, these factors work together to support hormone balance - yes, EVEN in perimenopause.

Before we take a closer look at how Food can ease our symptoms, let me share some of the guiding principles that are at the foundation of the Thrive Method for Hormone Balance, my signature method for returning vibrancy and balance to the body by addressing root causes of hormonal imbalances and using food to load the body with essential nutrients that allow women to THRIVE through the stages of menopause.

Principles to Thrive
Our bodies are:
- Resilient.
- Always guiding us.
- Designed to Thrive at all ages.

That's right. Contrary to popular belief, Menopause is NOT
The end of feeling good,
The end of happiness, or
The end of having a fun and active life.

In fact – the symptoms that are making you feel less than awesome, are an opportunity to turn your health around, make your symptoms fade away, and feel better than ever.

Remember these Principles:

Your body is RESILIENT.

I'm obsessed with the body's ability to heal, repair and bring itself to balance. When we understand what our bodies are asking for, we can provide what they need – *with FOOD* – to function the way they're designed to – with energy, happiness, flexibility, strength and passion.

I have seen people make remarkable shifts in their bodies with incredible results like: losing significant weight, getting themselves out of pain, making their hot flashes disappear, boosting their energy, sleeping through the night, clearing brain fog, getting rid of anxiety and more.

Remember – Your body is resilient and will gift you with incredible health when you gift yourself with prioritizing your physical, mental, and spiritual health.

Your body is always guiding you.

Women are very intuitive, especially when it comes to our bodies. When we cultivate this connection, we trust the answers within us and know that our bodies are always guiding us back to health.

If the body needs help, THE ONLY WAY IT HAS TO COMMUNICATE WITH US IS BY SYMPTOMS.

Let's embrace the paradigm that our symptoms are guiding us back to health rather than the outdated and fear-based belief that symptoms mean something is broken and needs to be fixed. When we adopt this more empowering truth – we appreciate all the signs and signals our body gives us so we can make choices that are best for OUR body to feel alive, vibrant and passionate about life.

Designed to THRIVE at ALL ages.

Yes – even through the years of perimenopause. The body is designed to be in balance. At the cellular level every innate function is performed with the intention of keeping the cell healthy, the surrounding tissues healthy, the organs and muscles and so on – all operating together to stay in balance.

Perimenopause is a gradual process that can take approximately 10 years. The reason this transition to menopause and beyond spans nearly a decade is because it is meant to be gradual, gentle and ease our bodies into a different state of lower hormone levels. Even though you may not be experiencing a smooth perimenopause right now, your body is resilient enough to come back to balance and minimize or even eliminate your symptoms.

The fastest way to get our cells the nutrients they are designed to utilize so they can perform their job(s) well, keep our hormones balanced, and ease our symptoms is to eat high quality nutrients. How else will our cells get the nutrients they need?

Foods and nutrients that support hormone balance.

Phytonutrients for Balance
Phytonutrients are vitamins, minerals and other beneficial compounds, like phytoestrogens, found abundantly in fruits, vegetables, nuts, seeds, and whole grains. Through the stages of menopause, they can play a crucial role in balancing

hormone levels and reducing inflammation. One group of phytonutrients, known as lignans, found in flaxseeds, sesameseeds, whole grains, and unprocessed soy, can mimic estrogen effects in the body (phytoestrogens), and studies have found they may ease hot flashes and other symptoms by reducing hormonal fluctuations.

Omega-3 Fatty Acids for Mood and Joint Pain
Omega-3 fatty acids are renowned for their anti-inflammatory properties and have been linked to improved mood and even heart health. As perimenopause can bring about mood swings, achy joints and sometimes skin inflammation, incorporating fatty fish like salmon, chia seeds, walnuts, and flaxseeds into the diet can offer relief. Omega-3s support brain function, help regulate emotions, and maintain cardiovascular health.

High Quality Proteins: Supporting Metabolism
As estrogen levels decline during the stages of menopause, women may experience changes in metabolism and have difficulty maintaining their weight. Incorporating high quality animal and plant-based protein sources such as beans, lentils, tofu, and quinoa can help support muscle maintenance, boost metabolism, and provide a sustained source of energy. Most women don't get enough protein - aim for about 20 g per meal. These proteins also contain essential amino acids that aid in hormone production and overall bodily functions.

Be sure to work with an expert to make sure your digestion is strong enough to break down these important proteins so you can reap the benefits!

Fiber: Regulating Digestion and Hormones

A diet rich in fiber offers numerous benefits for women navigating menopause. Fiber aids in digestion, prevents constipation, and can help regulate hormone levels by supporting healthy gut bacteria. Nuts, seeds, vegetables, fruits, legumes, and whole grains are excellent sources of dietary fiber that can promote hormonal balance and may ease symptoms like heavy periods, breast tenderness, mood swings, headaches and more.

Bitter Foods: Supporting Detoxification of Excess Hormones

Dark leafy greens, cruciferous veggies, legumes, bitter melon, coffee (be careful here) and raw cacao offer the benefits of the bitter taste which have been found to support the liver and digestion. The liver is responsible for detoxification of hormone disrupting toxins and even excess hormones like estrogen and cortisol. Bitter foods help the body digest fats, metabolize excess hormones, balance blood sugar, and ease symptoms like bloating and gas, indigestion, and cravings.

Mindful Eating: Cultivating a Positive Relationship with Food

Beyond the nutritional benefits, adopting a mindful approach to eating can greatly impact overall well-being during the phases of menopause. With so much emotion and judgement attached to food, part of using food as medicine is to practice releasing judgement and becoming the observer. Notice what foods make you feel good, and which ones make your symptoms worse. And then, take your power back by making choices that give you energy, clarity, and joy. Allow yourself to ride the waves of this journey with food and give yourself grace. Once you are clear on how you want to feel, you'll naturally begin choosing foods that help you feel that way more and more often. And when you want to have wine and cake occasionally, you'll let go of judgement and enjoy every sip and bite. It really is that simple.

Personalization and Professional Guidance

It's essential to recognize that every woman's experience of menopause is unique. While eating whole, nutrient dense foods more often will improve your hormone health, consulting with healthcare professionals and hormone balance experts is crucial. They will assess what foods will support YOUR body the most, and determine whether your body is absorbing and metabolizing these beneficial foods. Working with an expert can provide you with personalized guidance based on individual health conditions, lab results, functional testing, and your current symptoms.

Final Thoughts

The challenges that often accompany the transition to menopause don't have to get in the way of living a full, happy, active life. You can learn to be in tune with your body as you go through this transition phase, and let it guide you to what is best for YOUR body.

Your mission is to provide your body with the nutrients, love, rest, laughter, peace and movement it needs to keep your hormones balanced, and you feeling like your happy, energetic self again!

You've got this - and you can start harnessing the power of food today!

You've got the information, now it's time to TAKE ACTION. Download the **Free Ayurvedic Guide to Balanced Hormones.**

Journal Prompts:

Take a moment. Close your eyes. Take a deep breath. Get still and quiet in your mind. Now ask yourself, "What does my body need today?". Remain still and present and notice what comes up for you. Don't overthink it. Keep it simple. Write down what came through for you. Finally, find a way to honor your body's wisdom and messages that you wrote down in your journal. You've got this.

CHAPTER SIXTEEN
Regaining control of your mind and your body
by Geraldine Joaquim

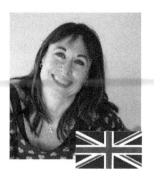

Bio: Before training as a hypnotherapist, I worked in international marketing. Unfortunately I found myself 'running on empty', which manifested in being high functioning but not really engaged, particularly with my growing family – there was just no spare capacity to do anything outside the routine and that's not much fun! I needed a change... So, in 2016 at the age of 46 I started training to become a Solution Focused Hypnotherapist.

Since then, I've helped numerous clients with a diverse range of issues, but I have found a particular interest in sleep disorders, women's health and menopause, and healthy weight loss.

In 2020 I was diagnosed with breast cancer which prompted me to explore non-HRT solutions to help support my own perimenopause symptoms, so I've been there/done that!

Business: Geraldine Joaquim
Website: www.geraldinejoaquim.co.uk

Life… it's stressful, isn't it? The constant demands on your time and attention, and then you add in hormonal fluctuations, the peri-rage or brain fog, and maybe feeling like the years are slipping away because menopause is like a curtain coming down on the first act called 'youth'.

It can feel like you're losing control of everything!

Don't despair! Yes, there are changes afoot, maybe lots of them, and not just in your body but in your mind too, how you see yourself, how others treat you, maybe feeling invisible, under-valued and taken for granted, assuming everyone else has got their lives sorted…

Let's rewind a bit though, start with what the menopause is all about.

One theory is that from an evolutionary perspective it makes sense for younger women to continue to ensure the survival of the species, with their stronger, healthier bodies able to withstand the rigours of pregnancy and childbirth, so nature just kind of gives up on us older ladies… After all, when females can no longer have babies, what use are they?? It's just not worth the energy investment so oestrogen and progesterone production plummets from 100% to just 2%.

And another theory is that older women are full of wisdom and have a greater capacity to support others. Studies in the 1960's suggest that menopause has a more functional reason than nature simply washing her hands of us – it's actually beneficial for the survival of the tribe not to produce children across generations at the same time, but instead older women can support their daughters in the rearing of their young. And it's interesting that there are only two other animal species known to go through menopause: killer whales and short-finned pilot whales. It's suggested that whales do this to focus their attention on the survival of their families rather than on birthing more offspring – not unlike humans.

And here's yet another theory – that menopause is our time to look after ourselves after decades of being there for everyone else, the raging hormones are actually bolstering your ability to say "No" after years of acquiescing. Maybe nature is actually giving us back our lives after all that child-rearing, cleaning, cooking, working and supporting everyone else…

Whichever theory you choose to ascribe to, without a doubt during peri- and on through menopause your hormones are in a huge state of flux and that impacts on how you feel, and the more you feel out of control, the more stressed and overwhelmed you become, it's a vicious cycle that feeds into itself.

So, how do you get the most out of this life stage especially when it can feel like everything is going south?

It all starts in your mind…

I just said to myself, "Cheer up, I've got loads to be happy about!" and it worked… said no one, ever.

Reframing is a powerful tool you can use to change the way you see things, and that in turn can help reduce your stress levels and even rebalance your hormones. When you think better, you feel better... and it becomes a positive cycle that helps you cope with whatever life (and menopause) throws at you.

So, I just have to think myself happy..?

Of course it's not that simple!

It's no good telling yourself to "buck up – woman up – get a grip" because you simply can't help how you feel; your emotional state happens to you, feelings are a response mechanism, but you can influence them by changing your:
- Thoughts, and/or
- Actions, and/or
- Environment

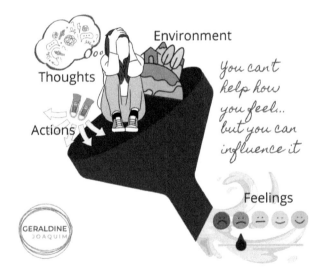

154

Let's face it, if you're sitting on the sofa in a dark and dingy room, watching rubbish tv and eating rubbish food, thinking rubbish thoughts about yourself, it's likely that you're going to feel a bit, well, rubbish.

So change something. It doesn't have to be big, just start with a small change in your thoughts, behaviour or environment, such as getting up off the sofa and making a cup of tea, or switching the tv off and reading a book, or clearing the rubbish off the table in front of you, or going outside to breathe some fresh air for 5 minutes. Then build on it day by day, add in another small change, it's called habit stacking and it supports you in making positive changes gently.

The easiest elements to change are behaviour and environment, what you're doing and where you are; simply by getting up and walking into another room or going outside you're doing both. For most people the hardest one is what's happening in your mind.

And that brings us back to reframing – your brain is constantly looking for evidence of the person you are, if you think of yourself negatively: I'm useless, I'm ugly, I'm old, I always feel terrible, these symptoms are going to last forever, no one loves me; then your brain rather helpfully focuses on those thoughts and gives you more of the same, a downward spiral of negativity that doesn't just affect your thoughts but it affects your physical health too.

Because you release cortisol when you feel bad or stressed, and cortisol upsets your hormonal balance: the more cortisol you have in your system, the less oestrogen and progesterone is produced. Nothing works in isolation, there's always cause and effect going on.

So, guess what? You feel worse, and that lack of oestrogen and progesterone is exacerbated, resulting in your symptoms ramping up even more.

Think of your attention like a torch beam, you can choose where you shine that beam of light. The more you focus on negative thoughts, the more negative thoughts you'll notice, but when you switch the polarity around and train it onto more positive things, you'll get more of the same.

At first it might feel a little awkward, that's because you've developed a habit of existing in a certain way and it takes conscious effort to make a new habit. Remember when you first learned to ride a bike or drive a car, you had to do all that 'mirror, signal, manoeuvre' deliberately from the conscious part of your brain until it became a habit, an action you have since done hundreds, thousands of times so you no longer have to think your way through it, it's become a subconscious action but you do still do it – unless you're a driver who has a long line of car crashes behind you every time you pull out into traffic!

The first step is developing your self-awareness:
- Notice the thoughts that are going through your mind

- Notice if you have any behaviours that may not make you feel great
- Notice if you've fallen into habits that no longer work for you
- Notice how you're feeling in relation to your environment.

Then think about what you want to do about any of it. Are there any small changes you want to make to your thoughts, actions, environment..? It might help you to keep a journal or just jot your thoughts down to keep some kind of record.

None of these things happen overnight, it takes time and patience to redirect your thoughts and change your behaviour but by doing it consistently you will start to notice a difference in how you feel.

When you start to reframe what's happening around you and within you, you're taking a mental step back which allows you to see the bigger picture, and then to choose how you respond instead of reacting in the same way you've always done, which isn't really helping you much.

And keep in mind that all your thoughts are merely your interpretation of how things are, they're not fact or necessarily true... a bit like deciding which of those menopause scenarios I mentioned earlier works for you.

Has nature discarded you like yesterday's old rag?

Or do you think there's a bigger plan that places you front and centre in shaping the next generation?

Or maybe you prefer to see this phase as a kind of re-birth, preparing you for the next part of your life as a strong and commanding presence, being the person you want to be instead of the person you happen to be?

By choosing how you perceive things, you're taking back control of your mind and also to some extent your body.

You probably won't be free of all the symptoms of menopause – let's be realistic here, there are real physical changes happening and you can't simply think yourself out of them – but you will have a greater capacity to cope, you'll feel calmer, more at peace with that's happening, and you'll find that those symptoms don't impact on you in quite the same way as they did before.

Stop struggling on your own, help is at hand... contact me now for a free no-obligation chat.
Quote 'perihub book' for 10% discount off your first session. It's time to get back to the real you.

Journal prompts:

How do you know you're on an even keel? (i.e. what are you doing/feeling that keeps you going/happy?)

What are the reg flags that tell you you're going off track? (i.e. not exercising, binge watching tv, eating unhealthy foods).

How do you know you've completely de-railed? (i.e. feeling de-motivated, letting negative thoughts take over, sleep issues).

Now, make a note of those activities, your environment and positive thoughts that keep you motivated, build your resilience and help you to stay in control.

CHAPTER SEVENTEEN
Should I Consider
Taking HRT?
by Dr Susanna Unsworth

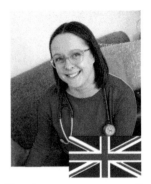

Bio: Hello! I'm Dr Susanna Unsworth. During my career I have dedicated time to developing my knowledge of women's health and am registered on the British Menopause Society Register of Menopause Specialists.

In the NHS, I work as a Specialist in Breast Medicine at Addenbrookes Hospital in Cambridge, supporting women after a breast cancer diagnosis, and as a Community Gynaecology Specialist GP in Essex.

In addition to my NHS roles, I run Cambridge Women's Health: a specialist online clinic for women who are facing challenges with menopause. I have developed a menopause supplement to offer a simple option for women looking for something to support themselves through the menopause transition: Meno8.

Business: Cambridge Women's Health
Website: www.cambridgewomenshealth.co.uk

Writing a chapter on HRT is quite a challenge. You could fill multiple books (and people have!) with information on HRT alone. Therefore, I am going to focus on discussing what I feel is important to understand when it comes to HRT – the regimes available, along with the risks and benefits it brings – so that you can make an informed decision about whether HRT is the right choice for you.

Should I consider taking HRT?

Current guidance from NICE (National Institute for Health and Care Excellence) is that HRT is used to alleviate symptoms of perimenopause and menopause. Therefore, if you are experiencing symptoms of perimenopause or menopause that are impacting on your quality of life, I would recommend you consider the potential for using HRT. Sadly, I often see women who are seriously struggling, and have been for some time, and HRT has not even been discussed. There may be factors in your own history that will affect how safe HRT is for you as an individual, but I believe all women should be given the opportunity to discuss this option and make an informed choice.

So, what is HRT?

This seems like a really sensible place to start!

The term HRT stands for hormone replacement therapy. Really, it is more accurate for us to refer to it as menopause hormone therapy (MHT), and you may find it described as this in a number of different resources. However, for this book I have opted to continue with the term 'HRT' as I feel that is what most people recognise.

HRT is a treatment given to relieve the symptoms of perimenopause and menopause, either by stabilising or replacing the changing hormone levels that occur during this phase in life. For those that experience menopause at a very young age, it is also considered a treatment to prevent the health implications of hormonal loss occurring too early. HRT generally consists of a form of oestrogen, with or without a progestogen. Generally, it is the oestrogen element that provides the symptom relief, along with the longer term health benefits too. The progestogen is used to provide endometrial (womb-lining) protection.

What are the different HRT regimes?

HRT comes in two main forms. It can either be oestrogen-only HRT, or combined HRT, which consists of an oestrogen plus a progestogen. Combined HRT is then further subdivided into either cyclical or continuous, depending on whether the progestogen is taken every day or in a cycle pattern.

How do I know which regime I need to take?

The simplest question to ask to decide which regime is needed is this: have I had a hysterectomy?

For those who have had a full hysterectomy, oestrogen-only HRT will usually be recommended (there are some situations where this may not be the case, such as those with a history of endometriosis, where it can be beneficial to also include a progestogen). However, for everyone else, which is likely to be most women, combined HRT is required.

The reason for this is that when a form of oestrogen is given on its own, it has an effect on the womb lining (endometrium), causing thickening. This increases the risk of developing cancer of the womb. Therefore, if you still have your womb, you need to be given a progestogen alongside the oestrogen to prevent this from happening: providing 'endometrial protection'.

When combined HRT is required, we then need to decide whether it should be taken in a cyclical or continuous pattern. Usually, this is based on whether or not you are still having periods. For those who have not yet gone 12 months without a period, we would usually initially offer a cyclical regime of HRT. This would mean you would continue to bleed on a monthly basis, although the bleeding is often triggered by the HRT itself. For those who have gone 12 months without a period (by definition they are then postmenopausal) we would offer a continuous regime. This regime should not cause any bleeding beyond the first 3-6 months after initiation.

However, this is not a hard and fast rule, and there may be reasons to choose a continuous regime in women who are still having periods, such as those who struggle with cyclical mood changes or migraines. It is also recommended to consider using a continuous regime in women who are naturally reaching the expected age of menopause, around age 51. If women do use a continuous regime and they are not quite postmenopausal, it can lead to erratic bleeding.

Choosing the right HRT product.

At my last count, there are well over 50 different options for HRT products currently available in the UK. That is great news as it means there are lots of choices of products to allow us to really individualise treatment.

Oestrogen can be given via the following routes: oral as a tablet, transdermal (through the skin) as either a gel, patch or spray, or even as an implant, although this is less readily available. There are also vaginal forms of oestrogen which are used to treat localised vaginal and urinary symptoms.

The progestogen element of HRT can also be given orally, either combined with the oestrogen in one tablet, or on its own, or as a transdermal combined patch. It can also be delivered directly into the endometrium using a hormonal intrauterine system, often referred to as the 'coil'. Some doctors may advise giving certain types of progestogen via the vaginal route if side-effects are an issue. However, there are currently no HRT products licensed to be used this way, so this should always be discussed with your prescribing doctor first.

The actual HRT products used should be based on your individual circumstances. There may be medical reasons why we would not recommend an oral form of oestrogen, such as a history of migraine with aura, or those with a family history of blood clotting issues. It may also be important to consider the need for contraception, as HRT does not generally offer this. You may also have personal reasons for wanting to choose a certain product. Many women are currently opting to use a form of HRT known as body identical. This means the hormones it contains are structurally the same as the natural hormones found in our body, although they are synthesised in the lab – this consists of oestradiol along with micronised progesterone. Data has shown that body identical HRT is associated with the lowest overall risk of breast cancer so it is often considered to be the gold standard option to begin with.

What are the benefits of HRT?
As with any treatment, it is important to have an understanding of the risks and benefits, so you can look at both sides of things before making a decision about whether it is right for you.

The biggest benefit that HRT provides is very effective relief from menopausal symptoms. This book is full of other advice and treatment options that you can also consider to support you through your menopause transition, but given the symptoms are a consequence of hormonal change, the most effective treatment is likely to be something that restores that hormone balance. For the vast majority of women, if the right HRT is chosen, it will be very effective at resolving their symptoms.

There are also other potential benefits that HRT can offer, particularly if it is started early in the menopause transition. HRT can have a beneficial effect on cardiovascular risk, and it has also been shown to prevent and reverse bone loss that occurs as a consequence of reduced oestrogen. It has also been suggested that HRT may have a role in the risk of dementia, although currently the data assessing this is conflicting. Whilst HRT is not currently recommended as a preventative treatment, it is important to take these additional benefits into account when weighing up your decision about using it.

What about the risks?

In my experience, the risk that most women worry about is breast cancer. Therefore, I feel that this is the risk that is important to address. Sadly, clinical studies from the past, which were often misrepresented in the media, have led to an over-exaggerated perception of the actual risk that HRT confers in relation to breast cancer. So here are a few points I often discuss with patients in my clinic to help them understand the level of risk:

- For women who experience menopausal symptoms early, using HRT up to the age of 50 is not associated with any increase in breast cancer risk. We are simply replacing hormones they should naturally have.
- Evidence has shown that when using oestrogen–only HRT, the risk of breast cancer does not appear to be any higher than that seen in women not taking HRT.
- In women aged 50-60, when using combined HRT, there is a small increase in the risk of being diagnosed with breast cancer when HRT is used for five years or more, but this risk is lower than the risk of drinking two units of alcohol per day or being overweight/obese.

In addition to breast cancer there are some other risks it is important to be aware of. The most significant is a type of blood clotting called venous thromboembolism. Oral oestrogen, and some synthetic progestogens, increase the risk of blood clotting. However, it has been shown that if oestrogen is delivered via the skin (transdermal), rather than as an oral treatment, there is no increase in clotting risk. In addition, the body-identical progesterone also has a much lower clotting risk. Therefore, in women who may have pre-existing risk factors for blood clotting conditions, or have a previous history of a blood clot themselves, transdermal body-identical HRT would be recommended.

There are also some potential cardiovascular risks associated with using HRT (again, these are considered lower with the body identical and transdermal preparations). There is an increased risk of heart attacks and strokes seen in women taking oral forms of HRT, which is noted to be more significant if HRT is started more than 10 years since natural menopause occurred, or in those aged over 60.

There have been some associations with endometrial cancer and ovarian cancer seen with certain forms of HRT. These risks are low, and the risk of endometrial cancer is significantly reduced by using appropriate progestogen treatment alongside oestrogen.

It is important to view these risks alongside the benefits of HRT: effective symptom control, along with potential cardiovascular, osteoporosis and even dementia benefits previously discussed. On balance, it is accepted that for most healthy women, the benefits of HRT significantly outweigh the risks.

What about side-effects?
Whilst we have mainly focused on the more serious risks associated with HRT, there are also some potential side-effects. Oestrogen can trigger nausea, breast tenderness and headaches. Progestogens are associated with stomach upset, bloating and also changes in mood. For many, these side-effects will resolve in the first few weeks. However, if things persist, changes to the HRT regime can be made and, in my experience, it is usually possible to find a preparation that will remove these side-effects.

Summary
This really has been a whistlestop tour of HRT and there are a million other things that I could talk about. If there is a take-home message I would like to share, it is that HRT can be considered by most women and it can be started when you are still having periods. The important thing is to balance the potential benefits against the risks for you as an individual, to allow you to make an informed choice about what will help you navigate through your own menopause journey.

To book a consultation, visit
cambridgewomenshealth.co.uk.

Learn more about the Meno8 supplements
via the QR code.

Notes:

CHAPTER EIGHTEEN
HRT or Natural -
Which One Is Best?
by Hannah Charman

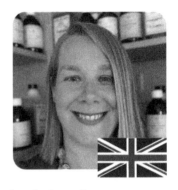

Bio: Hannah found herself beyond the help of mainstream medicine when she was just 14, and used a number of alternative treatments to recover from Chronic Fatigue Syndrome. She first trained in Reiki at the age of 16, and went on to qualify as a Medical Herbalist in 1999 following 4 years of intensive training. Since then Hannah has specialised in supporting women who can't or don't want to take HRT, combining prescribed herbal medicine with health coaching and advanced hypnotherapy into unique treatment programmes.

Hannah lives in Shropshire, UK with her partner and son, and enjoys coffee, gardening, and walks in the country.

Business: Physic Health
Website: www.physichealth.uk

If you're one of those ladies who's been advised against HRT, or you simply prefer a more natural approach, what other options are there? There are so many products, services and different offerings out there, sifting through them can become quite overwhelming, and can cost you a lot of time and money. So let's look at some tried and tested options, and see how they compare to HRT.

What Natural Options Are There?

I've worked in natural medicine for quite a long time now, and in my world we always look at menopause in the context of your overall health. Often we've put everyone else first for decades by the time we enter perimenopause, neglecting our own needs for sleep, rest, activity and good nutrition. It's not surprising then that I always suggest starting with upping the self-care. Regardless of which other treatments you may like to use in future, if you don't have the foundations of good health in place, it will impact your quality of life in the short and long term.

I don't want to focus on that too much here, but I will say that even small changes to your diet and lifestyle make a really big difference when it comes to self-care. We know for example that just 30 minutes of exercise a day can cut your risk of dementia by up to 40%. We know that minimising sugar, processed foods and carbohydrates not only helps you manage your weight in menopause, but reduces the inflammation linked to cancer, heart disease and brain degeneration later in life. Any little thing you can do is a big step in the right direction.

Herbal remedies also offer a great way through perimenopause, whether or not HRT is an option. They're what our ancestors would have used, and much of the world's population still rely largely on herbal medicines even now. The difficulty, again, is knowing which ones to take, especially if you've got other health issues besides menopause, or you're on other medication.

Should I look after myself or let someone else look after me?

I think you should let someone else look after you!

Why? Because if you're like most women, you'll have been putting yourself last for quite a long time now. If you're a mum or carer, family will have come first. If you're also a career woman, you've probably put working long hours first too. We all do it! But the problem is that the menopause transition is a big ask of the human body, and if you've skimped on sleep, nutrition, relaxation and/or exercise for decades, you're inevitably going to struggle. The other problem is that there are probably still a number of people depending on you to show up and function in whichever capacity they see you. How can you possibly do that if menopause has literally left you too exhausted to move?

Of course, there's an investment that comes with letting someone else to look after you, but if you can find the funds it's money well spent. Whether it's a weekly coffee and chat with the girls, a monthly massage, or some really intensive treatment, it's 100% worth it not just for your sake but for those around you as well.

If you're just noticing some subtle changes or mild symptoms, it's much easier to get by with self-care alone than if they've gone off the scale. Knowing what to do is one thing, but actually being able to do it is altogether different. It takes real effort to get up and exercise when you don't feel like it, or to choose a chicken salad over fish and chips when you're too tired to cook. So if your self-discipline isn't where it needs to be, find an accountability partner to work with.

What to look for in a practitioner

A lot of alternative therapies are not state regulated in the UK, so you need to do your own research before choosing a reliable practitioner. Here's a quick checklist to help you:
Ask how and where they trained, how long for and what qualification(s) they have.

- Ask what kind of ongoing learning they've done since qualifying.
- Find out if they have insurance, and are a member of a governing body.
- Ask to see copies of testimonials from their other patients/clients.

It's common for practitioners to ask for at least part payment for your appointment when they book you in.

How Do Natural Options Help Protect Me After Menopause?

It's important to know that there's no 'natural HRT' as such. Natural remedies are not going to top your body up with hormones which would naturally be in decline. What they will do is support your body as it moves through the process, calming the wild fluctuations in hormones and making the whole process much gentler. When you remember that you've created yourself from 2 cells into a perfect human, survived childhood, adolescence, adulthood, possibly pregnancy and birth and completed any repairs needed along the way, it's a bit easier to trust your body to do menopause too. Usually if we give ourselves the time, care and resources we need, we can sail through the menopause under our own steam. That's what we're doing with natural options.

Our health after menopause depends largely not just on how menopause itself goes, but how well we are in the decades leading up to that. Your menstrual health is an indicator of your overall health, and it's important to try and have normal, natural cycles for as long as possible if you want to protect your wellbeing into old age. That means choosing non-hormonal contraception, and seeking suitable treatment for any gynae conditions that might prevent you from having monthly periods.

At the time of writing, the British Menopause Society and governing bodies like the RCOG do not recommend using HRT as a means of protecting against dementia, osteoporosis or heart disease as there's insufficient evidence to support using it in this way.

Is Herbal Medicine A Good Alternative?

In my experience as a medical herbalist specialising in menopause, prescribed herbal medicines have a number of advantages over HRT. When I see a new patient for help with menopause, I take their entire medical history from birth to the present day, and put their symptoms in that context. That gives me a clear picture of what the underlying causes of any symptoms are likely to be, and which herbs we need to correct them. Occasionally I also notice symptoms which may not be perimenopause related, in which case I discuss them with the patient and recommend asking their GP for further tests to rule out other possible causes. It can be literally lifesaving.

Treatment is a three way partnership between me, my patient, and the herbs. Herbs are intelligent medicines working in an intelligent body, acting a bit like a mechanic tweaking and nudging the body's processes in a healthier direction. In my experience they can relieve symptoms just as quickly as HRT, but without any worries about shortages or side effects. The patient is always in control of their overall treatment, and if there are numerous symptoms, I ask her to prioritise which ones to start from. As each one subsides, we move onto the next and I change the prescription accordingly, so it's very versatile, and it's lovely for the woman to feel back more in control over her own body. As well as an internal mix to address the underlying causes, I might also use a sleep mix, herbal pessaries, or aromatherapy nasal inhalers to treat specific symptoms. When they feel completely well again, it's normal for my patients to wean slowly off their medicine altogether.

Seeing a medical herbalist is about far more than just taking medicine though. Often there are changes to be made in diet, sleep hygiene, exercise routines, or stress management which will help get the foundations of good health in place. That not only supports the herbs in their work, but helps to speed up the treatment process, and maintain optimum health post menopause too.

Despite herbal medicine only receiving 0.1 % of the global research budget, there's a surprising amount of research backing its use, especially when it comes to perimenopause. In the UK perimenopause is the only condition that GP's are allowed to recommend herbs for, because there's sufficient evidence. Some Oncologists also recognise that herbal medicine offers a safe and effective alternative to HRT for women who've had oestrogen receptive cancers.

To my knowledge there are no studies comparing HRT with herbs for perimenopause. There are studies backing the use of Sage in improving brain function and protecting against dementia post menopause. Likewise there are some indicating that Mexican Wild Yam stimulates the cells which build bone, and helps protect against osteoporosis. You can find out more by searching the Pubmed website.

The only downside to working with a medical herbalist is the cost, but perimenopause gives us a golden opportunity to transform your physical, emotional and even spiritual health, and you're totally worth the investment.

How perimenopausal are you, and what might work best for you at this stage? Click through on the QR code and scroll down on the page to complete my free questionnaire and find out:

Notes:

CHAPTER NINETEEN
Hormone Testing during Perimenopause:
A Deep Dive
by Dr Tanya McEachern

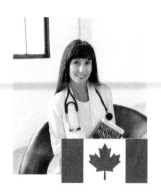

Bio: Dr. Tanya McEachern is a renowned Naturopathic Doctor with a dedicated passion for holistic women's health. Drawing from years of experience and expertise, she brings a unique perspective on natural and integrative approaches to menopause. Her work has helped illuminate the path for over 400 women seeking balance and well-being during this significant phase of life.

Business: Dr. Tanya McEachern, ND
Website: www.TanyaMcEachern.com

"In the chapter 'Hormone Testing During Perimenopause: A Deep Dive', readers are guided through the intricate world of hormone fluctuations that occur during perimenopause. This comprehensive exploration demystifies the process and significance of hormone testing, offering clear insights into why it's pivotal for understanding and managing this transitional phase. With expert advice and detailed explanations, this chapter is a must-read for anyone seeking to grasp the nuances of their changing hormonal landscape."

Perimenopause, the transition phase leading up to menopause, is a significant and, at times, challenging stage in a woman's life. It's a time when a woman's body begins to make less of the hormones that govern the reproductive system (oestrogens & progesterone), marking the gradual end of her fertility period. However, this hormonal shift isn't merely about fertility; it affects a woman's entire system, including other important hormones, often bringing about a myriad of symptoms.

Understanding these hormonal changes is paramount in managing perimenopause symptoms and ensuring a smoother transition. A key tool in this understanding is comprehensive hormone testing, which evaluates levels of key hormones such as estradiol, progesterone, testosterone, cortisol, and dehydroepiandrosterone (DHEA). Of the various testing methods available, urine and saliva tests are often most favoured due to their non-invasiveness, convenience, and capacity to accurately measure hormone metabolites in a way that serum testing cannot. In my practice, before prescribing any hormone replacement therapy or herbal remedies, I always run a comprehensive hormone test for my peri-menopausal patients.

Estradiol

Estradiol, one form of oestrogen, is a critical hormone for women. It plays a vital role in managing the menstrual cycle and maintaining the health of tissues such as those in the breasts, bones, brain, heart, and reproductive system. During perimenopause, estradiol levels can fluctuate wildly, eventually declining. This change can lead to a host of symptoms such as hot flashes, irregular periods, sleep disturbances, mood swings, and vaginal dryness.

To manage symptoms associated with a decline in estradiol, hormone therapy (HT) can be a possible solution. This treatment involves supplementing the body's declining hormones with synthetic or natural versions. My preferred treatment is Bio-Identical hormone replacement therapy containing a combination of estradiol and estriol, tailored to a particular woman's levels. This helps mitigate unwanted side effects like blood clots, stroke, and certain types of cancer. Non-hormonal treatments and lifestyle modifications, such as exercise, a balanced diet, and mind-body therapies, can also be effective, and are usually added to any treatment plan.

Progesterone

Progesterone, another crucial hormone in women's reproductive health, prepares the uterus for potential pregnancy following ovulation and helps maintain early pregnancy. However women have progesterone receptors in many other places too, such as the brain and the breasts. While progesterone helps counterbalance oestrogen's effects, it has value to help with symptoms like insomnia and anxiety as well. With the onset of perimenopause, progesterone levels often decline as the frequency of ovulation decreases. Symptoms of low progesterone include heavier or more frequent periods, mood swings, sleep disturbances, and low libido.

Salivary or urinary hormone testing can help gauge progesterone levels in the body. If an imbalance is detected, treatments can include progesterone therapy, using synthetic progestins or bioidentical progesterone (my preference). It's important to note that these treatments can come with side effects such as bloating, headaches, mood changes, and breast tenderness, but these are often dose related. Non-hormonal treatments and lifestyle modifications can also be effective in managing symptoms.

Testosterone

Testosterone, often thought of as a 'male' hormone, is actually incredibly important for women's health. It plays a role in maintaining bone and muscle mass (weight maintenance), and contributes to a healthy libido. In perimenopause, testosterone levels may decline, resulting in symptoms like fatigue, reduced sex drive, and loss of muscle tone.

Salivary or urinary hormone tests can be used to measure testosterone levels in women. Treatments for low testosterone can include testosterone replacement therapy, but as with all hormone treatments, it should be administered and monitored carefully to prevent side effects, which can include acne, hair loss, and voice deepening. Because of this, in my practice I prefer to use more natural approaches to boost testosterone levels, such as a diet rich in protein, zinc; strength training; and herbs such as Tribulus terrestris.

Cortisol

Cortisol, often dubbed the 'stress hormone,' is integral to our body's response to stress. It also helps regulate metabolism and inflammation and helps maintain blood sugar levels. During times of chronic stress or significant life changes like perimenopause, cortisol levels can become imbalanced, leading to symptoms like fatigue, difficulty sleeping, weight gain, and mood disorders.

Salivary or urinary testing is particularly useful for measuring cortisol, as it allows for multiple daily readings, providing insight into the hormone's natural rhythm throughout the day. Based on symptoms, it is impossible to tell whether cortisol is too high or too low. Neither scenario is good; we need our cortisol levels to be just right, with a proper daily rhythm (moderate upon waking, highest around noon, moderate around 3PM, low at bedtime).

Treatment for cortisol imbalance often involves lifestyle modifications such as stress management techniques, exercise, a balanced diet, and adequate sleep. Treatments differ greatly depending on whether we're trying to increase cortisol, or decrease it. For example, intense exercise helps to boost cortisol; we would want to avoid this in someone who is cortisol deficient. In more severe cases, medication under the guidance of a healthcare provider may be necessary, but generally cortisol responds well to natural remedies.

DHEA
DHEA is a hormone produced by the adrenal glands that serves as a precursor to other hormones, including oestrogen and testosterone. It has numerous roles, including boosting the

immune system, aiding in the production of other hormones, maintaining muscle mass, and improving mood and libido. During perimenopause, DHEA levels may decline, contributing to fatigue, a decrease in bone or muscle mass, and a lowered sex drive. DHEA and testosterone have many similarities in terms of symptoms they cause, however their function is quite different.

Saliva or urine tests can accurately measure DHEA levels. If low levels are detected, DHEA supplementation could be a potential treatment. It's important to note that DHEA supplementation should be carefully monitored due to potential side effects, including hair loss, acne, and mood changes.

Why saliva or urine?

All the hormones listed above are steroid-type hormones, and they have their action at the tissue level within the body. Blood primarily serves as a transportation medium for these hormones, ferrying them to different parts of the body where they act. Therefore, testing blood levels may not provide an accurate picture of what is occurring at the tissue level, where these hormones have their effects. It's akin to assessing the traffic flow on a highway without understanding the activities in the cities that the highway connects.

Moreover, hormone secretion is often pulsatile or cyclical, meaning the levels can fluctuate significantly throughout the day. These fluctuations are more pronounced in the blood than at the tissue level, leading to potential misinterpretations of hormone status if only blood levels are measured. For instance, a blood sample taken during a peak secretion time may incorrectly suggest excessively high hormone levels, while one taken during a trough may inaccurately indicate a deficiency.

In addition, if the blood being tested is venous blood – blood that is returning to the heart after supplying various body tissues – it has already offloaded its hormone cargo into the tissues. Thus, the hormone levels detected might be lower than the actual quantity delivered to the tissues, potentially resulting in underestimation of hormone activity.

For these reasons, many experts advocate for urine or saliva testing, which better reflects tissue-level hormone activity and can more accurately diagnose hormonal imbalances. These testing methods can also provide valuable insights into the efficacy of hormone-related treatments, helping to fine-tune therapeutic strategies. Understanding these distinctions is crucial in accurately interpreting hormone tests and developing appropriate treatment plans.

Understanding hormone levels during perimenopause is an integral part of managing the transition and mitigating troublesome symptoms. Through salivary or urinary testing, healthcare providers can gain valuable insights into a woman's hormonal health, enabling personalised treatment plans. While it can be tempting to aim to restore hormone levels to their youthful peak, the goal should be to achieve a balance that promotes overall wellbeing. As always, it's crucial to discuss your symptoms and concerns with a healthcare provider that you trust to determine the best course of action for you.

Love this chapter? If you're a woman in your 30s 40s, or 50s, you might be experiencing peri-menopausal symptoms. Get Dr. Tanya's FREE e-guide to help answer some of your burning health questions - don't miss out!

Journal prompts:

1. If you were to monitor one symptom of perimenopause daily, what would it be? Note down any patterns or changes over the next month.

2. Identify and list three aspects of your health or body for which you're grateful today.

3. Write down any lingering questions or concerns about hormone testing. How can you seek answers?

4. Before reading this chapter, what were your beliefs or assumptions about hormone testing? Have they changed?

5. List three things you plan to do or discuss with your healthcare provider after reading this chapter.

"Embrace menopause as a natural chapter in your story of womanhood. It's not the end of your vitality, but a transition towards a new depth of wisdom and health. Listen to your body, nourish it right, move with intention, and remember, every sunrise brings a new beginning." – Dr. Tanya

CHAPTER TWENTY
I is for Inflammation, Insulin Resistance and Finding the I in Perimenopause
by Toni Chambers

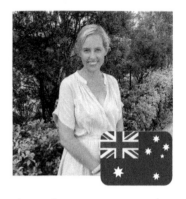

Bio: Toni is a passionate Australian clinical nutritionist who advocates for women's and children's health. Perimenopausal herself, Toni is facing many of the same challenges that you are, and has developed a 12-week program that has proven results for completely turning around the health of those who participate. Known for providing empathic and understanding one-on-one support, Toni helps participants devise an individualised plan.

Business: Healthy Midlife Woman Program
Website: https://www.tonichambers.com/

Understand what inflammation is and why it is driving so many symptoms we experience; understand how our hormonal changes make insulin resistance more likely and the role it plays in driving inflammation and weight gain. And lastly, see perimenopause through the lens of opportunity, a chance to get to know ourselves and adopt new lifestyle and dietary habits to support a healthy second life stage.

The world "inflammation" is bandied around without us really understanding what it means. Yet it is at the root of all chronic health conditions. Don't get me wrong we need inflammation, it is a very important response in the body. Acute inflammation is protective – if a virus or bacteria enters your body or if you injure yourself, like cutting your finger – your immune system responds by sending cells called cytokines to trap the pathogen and eventually remove it, or begin the process of healing the injury. This process is responsible for the redness, swelling, heat, pain and loss of function often associated with an injury.

The problem with inflammation is when it becomes chronic or continues even when the danger or injury is long gone. Chronic inflammation can happen in any part of our bodies and is often systemic, meaning our whole body is inflamed. But as Hippocrates said," All disease begins in the gut." So let's start there.

There are many causes of inflammation in our gastrointestinal tract – medications; a diet rich in sugars, processed foods, red meat and low in fibre rich fruits, vegetables and whole grains; altered gut bacteria caused by a poor diet and exacerbated by gut pathogens; and stress. All of these factors lead to the development of intestinal permeability or leaky gut. The cells of our small intestine are held together by tight gap junctions, but due to constant insults from our diet and lifestyle, they become looser and looser. The reason this is important is that an intact intestinal lining does not allow food particles, bugs, toxins from the environment, or the liver's breakdown products into our blood stream, but a leaky gut lining does.

Since these things are not meant to be in our blood stream, the immune system mounts an inflammatory response to rid the body of the "danger". This appears in the body as bloating, gas, diarrhoea, food sensitivities and fatigue, just to name a few. When some of the gut bacteria and their toxins enter the blood stream, the inflammatory response becomes systemic.

This is relevant for two reasons. Firstly, over time inflammation is the cause of weight gain that will not shift. The second builds on the first: in perimenopause oestrogen levels fluctuate. In the early part of the menopausal transition, your periods can be regular, proceeding to regular and light, short periods, right through to 60 days between periods until menopause is achieved. The overall shift however, is towards lower levels of oestrogen. Progesterone is in decline from the early stages of perimenopause. Both of these hormones have anti-inflammatory effects on the body which means we lose two of our biggest anti-inflammatory protectors and therefore, protection from weight gain (and many other chronic diseases).

The next "I" word is insulin resistance and it is intricately linked to inflammation. A short lesson in what insulin is: when we eat carbohydrates, our pancreas releases insulin that essentially knocks on the doors of our cells to let the glucose in. Our cells then use glucose to make energy. When we eat too many carbohydrates, usually in the form of sugar (lollies, soft drinks, chocolate, cakes, etc) over decades, our body is constantly releasing insulin and eventually the cell's doorman gets tired of listening to insulin. The pancreas releases more and more insulin (it is essentially shouting at the doorman!) until eventually the doorman will not open the door no matter how much insulin is knocking. This is called insulin resistance. Your cells are resistant to insulin's signals.

Bear with me while I bring all the pieces of the puzzle together. Remember oestrogen? Well, it performs many functions in the body as we begin to discover in perimenopause as we are starting to lose it. Isn't that always the way? You never know what you've got until it's gone! And oestrogen is no exception. Another role it plays in our body is removing glucose from the blood and therefore improving insulin sensitivity. It does this by improving glucose uptake into muscle cells and suppresses glucose production in the liver. More glucose in the blood leads to more insulin until eventually, insulin resistance develops. No matter what you do when you have insulin resistance, or even high levels in the blood, you cannot lose weight. You can eat small amounts and exercise all day, and the weight will not shift.

Higher insulin levels signal the body to store fat, especially around the abdominal area where many women in perimenopause experience weight gain. This type of fat is called visceral fat as it is stored around the internal organs, such as the liver, making it fatty. But more importantly, this fat is metabolically active, releasing inflammatory cytokines. Now, not only do we have high insulin levels in the blood, (and remember when this occurs, you cannot lose weight), but we have systemic inflammation which also leads to weight gain.

Another contributing factor in perimenopause is there are low levels (thought to be due to declining oestrogen) of adiponectin which increases insulin sensitivity.

Then there is a vicious cycle: As visceral fat increases inflammatory cytokines, adiponectin declines further and causes more insulin resistance which causes more weight gain and more inflammatory cytokines to be released. All of this equals more weight gain and an inability, no matter what we do, to lose it since insulin is a fat storage hormone.

One more point about abdominal weight gain, and that is stress…when we are under stress, our adrenal glands release cortisol to mobilise the body to run away from the proverbial tiger. But these days, there is no tiger, and stress is everywhere all the time. It's chronic. Cortisol too, is a fat storage hormone. It keeps glucose in the blood ready to be used for energy to run away from our tiger. This increases insulin and we know how that story goes. It also slows our metabolism down.

Women at this time are usually under chronic stress – they may be hitting the peak of their careers, still caring for teenage children, older parents and trying to deal with a major body and life change. If you are eating less and killing yourself on the treadmill at the gym and wondering why it isn't helping you lose weight, it's because these two factors INCREASE stress on the body and with declining progesterone, we have less stress resilience. Can you see now why energy in and energy out doesn't work? Weight loss and health now requires a more individualised approach.

This leads me to my final "I" word, finding the "I" in perimenopause. Weight gain is the number one gripe that women have during this time, and it is completely understandable. We align weight with self confidence. As we feel the pounds gradually increase, with everything we have ever tried in the past, now no longer working, it seems like this is our fate. But no, it is not.

And yes, I understand how important weight is and I also understand how difficult this time of life is, with all of its changes and symptoms and pressures. But believe me when I say, this time is a gift. Yes, you read correctly, it's a gift that men are not privileged enough to receive. For you who are experiencing debilitating anxiety, hot flushes, night sweats, depression, hives, weight gain and brain fog I see you, please don't stop reading. It's a gift because we are being given an opportunity to change our diet, lifestyle and mindset, and to find ourselves. Many of us, me included, get to this age and realise we don't know who we are. Every single post menopausal woman says it's the best time of their lives. Why? They know who they are, what they are prepared to do and what they aren't, who gives them energy and who drains them of energy. But these are the women who put in the hard yards. They took that class and worked out it wasn't for them; they sank into how they felt when their boundaries were crossed and learnt how best to assert them. These are our role models.

We have the choice to look deeply at ourselves and do a stocktake of our lives. What are we doing that no longer serves us? What habits, foods, alcohol, relationships, and jobs can we change. Most of all it's time to look in the mirror without averting our eyes and say, "I'm proud of you for everything you've been through and for how far you've come. What do you need now to live in health?" Your body knows the answer, all you have to do is listen.

I have a 12-week flagship program for women where we get to the bottom of underlying health issues and develop an individualised diet and lifestyle plan to thrive in mid-life that does not involve meal plans or restrictive eating.

Click on the QR code to book a 20-30 minute free discovery call.

Notes:

"The soul always knows how to heal itself. The challenge is to silence the mind."

CHAPTER TWENTY ONE
Just say No! - "Gatvol"
by Kirsten Alberts

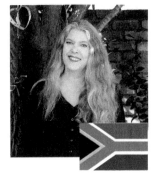

Bio: I am a Support and Trauma Counsellor specialising in identifying and breaking toxic patterns.

Business: Kirsten Alberts Counselling
Website: www.kirstenalberts.co.za

Maybe you're not just overworked, underpaid, and underappreciated. Maybe you're "Gatvol"

There is this saying in Afrikaans: "Gatvol". Loosely translated, it means "fed up". But, when the speaker uses this word, the listener Stops Breathing. Because by the time this marvellous word makes its appearance, the speaker is not simply "fed up", she is LIVID. Irritated beyond all comprehension. Over it. Done. Directly translated, "gat" means hole, and "vol" means full. Literally, so infuriated, her arse has had enough. Gatvol of the laundry nobody else seems to know how to do. Gatvol of the mess everyone knows how to make, but is incapable of even noticing. Gatvol of useless colleagues, needy neighbours, and bitchy in-laws. Gatvol of being overworked, underpaid, and unappreciated. All the things we did without complaint for decades, suddenly seem so irritating that just one more pile of laundry might actually be our undoing. (Or our family's).

Why?

As girls, and later as women, we have a set timeline. As little girls we are taught to be sweet, pretty, and ever helpful. We are expected to play nicely, have lots of other sweet, helpful friends, do well at school, and wear our ballet shoes with a smile, while our beaming mommies and daddies nod their approval. Up next on the timeline is our education. We are told that careers in altruism are what's best, so we enter institutions that will hone our skills, and we work diligently to make our parents and professors proud. When we enter the workforce, we repeat the process. We go above and beyond for our bosses and colleagues, making ourselves indispensable, so that our usefulness and tirelessness is rewarded. Next on the timeline is romance.

Our mothers and grandmothers have prepared us our whole lives for that walk down the aisle, and "we're not getting any younger, you know". So we sift through the hordes of boys within our radar. Boys that need to be smart, successful, and handsome, from good families, who will take care of us and our future children, and we pick one to present to our family.

Once we get the nod, we march down the aisle into wedded bliss, and onto the next item on the timeline: Settling Down. We buy a house, decorate it, and once we've filled it with furniture, we start filling it with children. Turns out, houses, furniture, and children come with hefty price tags, so we do everything we can to support our hardworking husbands. We delight in our happy children, so we do everything in our power to see them thrive. They need us to nurture, nourish, scold them and guide them, and even with the endless rounds of laundry, meals, and soccer practices, it feels good to be needed. So we keep going until our husbands are prosperous, and we see our kids becoming more and more independent.

Whelp, time for the next item on the timeline. So what is it? What's next? We check the timeline again. Sweet, agreeable daughter. Check. Education and career in approved field. Check. Marriage, house, children. Check, check, check. Where the hell is the rest of the timeline? The first 20 years we spent doing what our parents expected. The next 20 years goes on doing what our husbands and children expect. What are we expected to do for the next 20? With no one to tell us what is expected, no one to need us to feed them, or support them, or drive them god knows where, we feel completely rudderless. We've come to the end of our timeline and there's not even a cheap plastic participation prize? Because that's just it. No one hands out prizes for doing what is expected. Whether it's our hormones, our age, our experience, or all of the above, suddenly, doing what is expected doesn't seem very appealing anymore. In fact it's become downright infuriating. We've spent 40-odd years doing exactly what we're told, and now that we have, our timelines are over? No wonder we're annoyed. And well, GATVOL.

So what DO we do now? Well, we do whatever we want. We embrace our gatvol, ignore what everybody else thinks, and do whatever it is that WE expect will make US happy. All the times in the last 20 years we were expected to calm down and smile in case we were accused of "being on our periods", now that they're nearly over, we're expected to calm down lest we're accused of being "menopausal"? Good grief. The upside of our depleting oestrogen, is assertion. Revel in it.

We are not manifestations of other people's expectations. We are not our looks, or our boobs, or our figures, or our spotless floors. We are our experiences, talents, uniqueness, wisdom, and character. We are our sense of humour, our resilience, and our courage. We are the way we laugh, and love, and protect, and create. And we're going to spend the next 20-odd years writing our own damn timeline. Let's Get Gatvol. We've certainly earned it.

Email me at: info@kirstenalberts.co.za

Journal prompts:

What are the unnecessary things I do for other people that make me feel needed?

Tick the ones that can be reallocated, or scrapped altogether.

Do I know what I want to be "when I grow up"?

Partnerships and children aside, what fulfils me?

What changes can I make to do more of what fulfils me, versus what is expected of me.

Your Story Matters.

CHAPTER TWENTY TWO
Kindful Communication:
How to be Heard in the
Ways You Need
by Jo Jones

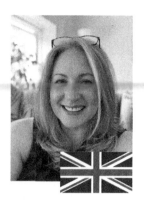

Bio: Jo Jones is The Peri Mind-Medicine Woman, an award-winning therapist, mindfulness teacher and perimenopause coach. She focuses on helping women to understand and recognise their thought processes, remove some of the scariness, dissolve shame gremlins, and hush their anxiety, to create a more self-compassionate and thriving version of themselves, on their empowered peri pathway.

Jo lives in the west country, near Bristol, UK with her partner, Jack, and their three over-affectionate dogs. She loves to bake bread, knit socks and is happiest with a large coffee, sunglasses on her head, walking in flip flops on a Cornwall beach.

Business: Hush TheraCoaching
Website: https://sleek.bio/johush

Perimenopause: a word that, for almost all of us, evokes a whirlwind of emotions and physical symptoms that sometimes feel overwhelming. And a particularly poignant challenge during this life phase is the act of communication, especially expressing our most intimate feelings and needs.

The Perimenopausal Communication Challenge

"Why, during perimenopause, does communication suddenly feel like I'm scaling Everest without an oxygen mask?"

Hormonal surges and fluctuations play a key role here. They bring with them a host of symptoms: rage, anxiety, brain fog, confusion, and the painful feelings of 'betrayal' by our changing bodies. Add to this an identity crisis as we grapple with the dawning of a new life phase, and it's no wonder finding the right words becomes more than challenging.

"During one particularly challenging evening, with a mix of hormonal surges and the stress of a long day, I found myself snapping at my partner over something trivial – the loading of the dishwasher! Suddenly, those saucepans on the top shelf and the glasses stacked in the bottom rack had me flipping my Tupperware lid! It wasn't just the fatigue talking; it was the culmination of feeling misunderstood, unheard, and isolated in my perimenopausal journey." - Why?!

Our fabulous brain, evolved over millennia to protect us, doesn't always get it right. Especially during this phase of life. Its main aim? Keeping us safe. However, amidst the hormonal tornado of perimenopause, this 'safety brain' can often misfire and do its job a bit too well. Responding to dangers and threats that it picks up on. That amygdala (our inner alarm button) going off, in a high-alert mode to everything that it senses as a problem. It can make us feel as though we're locked in a fortress, where our experiences are ring-fenced, isolated, leading to an overwhelming sensation that 'nobody understands us.'

Compounding this, us British women often indulge in a classic pastime: giving ourselves a bloody hard time. We berate ourselves for our feelings, for the angry words we might have spat out in frustration, or the tears shed in confusion. Now, more than ever, it's time to put the kettle on, take a deep breath, and pour ourselves a generously large cup of self-compassion.

This communication block is nothing you are doing wrong. Your feelings are not wrong. What we need here is some 'Kindful Communication'

Non-Violent Communication: A Beacon in the Fog

Enter 'Non-Violent Communication' (NVC), a mindfulness-based approach that feels like a breath of fresh air during the stuffy, disorienting swirly fog of perimenopause. Developed by Marshall Rosenberg, NVC aids us in expressing ourselves in a manner that's both compassionate and empowering.

"Much like many other women, I too walked that confusing labyrinth of perimenopause. There were days when I'd stare at my reflection, grappling with unfamiliar emotions, questioning my own reactions, and wondering why I felt so out of sync with myself."

Let me be really clear here – I'm not suggesting you were violent beforehand; it's just the name of this approach. I prefer to use the term 'Kindful' - Here's how it works.

Let's break it down:
1. **Feeling:** Start by expressing how you feel - Not a thought, but a genuine emotion. For example, I am feeling overwhelmed, I am feeling fatigued, I am feeling irritated. (Always identifying the feeling rather than pinning it to our identity - e.g. I am angry)

2. **Need:** Identify what you need or value, that's causing this feeling - Things like, feeling more valued, included, visible, more free time, wanting greater equality of work/chores, needing more balance or equity in decision making etc.

3. **Request:** Clearly ask what you'd like to happen – clear, concise, calm.

Maybe it's a quicker, more immediate ask; "Please could we load the dishwasher with the glasses at the top and fill it from the back?" – Ok, I know that was my experience.

Or "I would like to have a conversation about how we can make our big decisions differently – are you open to that?",

"When 'x' happens, I feel 'y' and I'd like to talk that through with you to find another way together – can we set a time to talk it over?"

4. **The Why:** Explain why this matters to you. You are allowed to have things matter to you! Explain how the changed outcome will help you and what it might change for you... and the other person.

The Power of Being Heard

Using Kindful NVC, we transform volatile emotions into honest, clear expressions of our needs. The beauty of this technique lies in its simplicity and mutual respect. It fosters understanding, reducing friction and resentment. Being truly 'heard' has an almost magical restorative power, providing validation, empathy, and connection.

It was during one of my own quests for clarity, as part of my Mindfulness Teacher training that I first encountered Non-Violent Communication. Initially sceptical, I decided to give it a go in my life, and the ripple effects it had on my interactions were profound. I felt like I had discovered a language that both my heart and mind understood.

Now, before you think, "Sounds lovely, Jo, but a bit pie in the sky for me," remember, like all skills, it simply takes a little bit of practice. And believe me, the outcomes are well worth the effort. The first time I employed NVC in a conversation with a close friend, the response was nothing short of illuminating. She paused, looked at me, and said, 'I never realised you felt this way, Jo.' That acknowledgment, that simple act of being heard, felt like a balm to my chaotic emotions.

I now incorporate this 'being heard' into my Women's Mind Medicine Circles as a healing tool – it's incredibly powerful.

Let's Try It Out

Imagine you're utterly worn out from the daily grind, the perimenopausal symptoms are wreaking havoc with you, and you feel the household chores are disproportionately landing on your shoulders. You want to discuss redistributing tasks with your partner, or even your teens.

Old way: "You never help around the house! I have to do everything, and you don't ever seem to care how I feel!"

Using NVC:
1. Feeling: "I'm feeling overwhelmed and exhausted lately."
2. Need: "I need a more equitable division of our household responsibilities, especially considering the physical and emotional toll of my perimenopausal symptoms."
3. Request: "Would you be open to discussing how we can share the chores more evenly?"
4. The Why: "It's important to me because I value our partnership, and I believe this will bring more balance for us both, and harmony to our home."

See the difference? The second approach opens the door for a constructive dialogue rather than laying blame.

Perimenopause is undeniably challenging. Yet, with tools like Kindful NVC, we can experience navigating these waters with grace, understanding, and genuine connection. As you find yourself at the cusp of this new life chapter, remember: your voice deserves to be heard, your feelings acknowledged, and your needs addressed.

As I integrated these communication techniques into my life, I found that not only did my professional interactions improve, but my personal relationships deepened, becoming more authentic and grounded. It wasn't an overnight transformation by any means, but each day brought with it a little more clarity and understanding. It was a practical, solid beacon during the bumpy storms of perimenopause.

Embrace kindful communication and watch as it not only transforms your relationships but also fortifies the connection with your evolving self. It's like a little dollop of mind medicine magic that could help you feel empowered, and just a little bit proud of yourself too.

Get more access to peri help with me in the HushPeri® Hub:

Reflection Points:

What needs am I noticing right now, that could use a conversation?

What do I want the outcome to be?

And imagining I've had this Kindful conversation, what feels different on the other side?

"Owning our story and loving ourselves through that process is the bravest things that we will ever do" – *Brené Brown*

CHAPTER TWENTY THREE
Your Midlife Guide to Smashing your Second Act: Visit 5 "Must Experience" Landmarks to Guide you to Lifelong Wellbeing by Sophia Cleverly

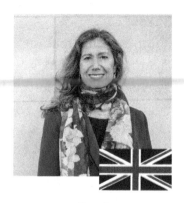

Bio: Sophia has worked in the wellbeing space for the past 10 years. Sophia is a certified life coach, having trained with The Co-Active Training Institute. Sophia is also a qualified Happiness Facilitator with training in Neuroscience and Positive Intelligence and seeks to coach women to recognise their unique values and leadership strengths to transcend their limitations and consciously create and live lives they love. Before becoming a mother, Sophia lived internationally, studied Greek and French at Oxford University and then worked as a producer in film and television which has given her an understanding of high pressure working life. Sophia lives in Oxfordshire with her husband Jesse, her three children - and her dog Ozzy!

Business: Sophia Cleverly Coaching: Life Coaching and Mentoring for Women navigating Midlife
Contact: The Happy Place Practice - sophiacleverlycoaching @gmail.com
Insta: @sophiacleverly

Summary

Things sometimes get worse before they get better – the caterpillar turns to goo before it transforms into the prized beauty of the butterfly. In the same way that each morning begins the night before, our midlife- and menopause-transition offer us the opportunity to learn how to look after our wellbeing like never before. What if all the symptoms were signs to help us figure it all out, so we can live longer, happier, healthier, and more authentic, purposeful lives?

Visit 5 "must experience" landmarks with me, your midlife travel guide.

Hey wonderful midlife woman, midlife warrior, midlife wanderer... allow me to be your travel guide in this part of your journey. I am going to make sure you visit 5 "must experience" midlife landmarks here. I see you walking down the midlife highway already, it is a road you have never encountered before but you have heard about it, read about it, watched others walk it; you have some ideas about what it might look like, feel like, sound like further down this road; you don't know much but let me tell you one thing for sure – there is no return.

You are heading into midlife. You are reading this so I am assuming that you are wanting to improve something or to better prepare yourself for the continuation of the journey. I am with you now if you will allow me to guide you. Imagine that there are some magic taliswomen or skills that you can pick up, right now in each of these 5 destinations I will lead you to. You will be able to practise with them and they will serve you on your journey, no matter where you come from, who you have been, what has happened to you. They will serve you moving forward and can shape your reality in your best interest from now on. Because, no matter what your story has been, you get to write the next part.

The tools I offer you below are the fruits of my own labour of love through the perimenopause birth canal to surface as the best version of me yet, as well as those of the women I help - women just like you navigating the bumpy terrain of perimenopause and midlife. Come and explore these five "must visit destinations" at this often uncertain and challenging landscape which can, as I am sure you are aware, last a long while until we reach the Promised Land of Second Spring or Post Menopause, when apparently it all gets better. Marvel at the outset that womenfolk have "done this" for centuries upon centuries and also that certain animals go through this integral transition.

Never have we known as much about it as we do now and yet also realise how many women have suffered before us and how many of us are also still suffering on . At this point in time, we have had enough of pretending it is okay to suffer on. I know you know this because you are here. So take my hand – it's your time. Let's walk together and step into a new story of empowerment.

Stop A: Awareness Archipelago.
Self-awareness is your map. Awareness of yourself as well as awareness of symptoms you might be encountering and ways

you can support yourself. To be self-aware means to know yourself. In your 40s and beyond, this will entail checking in with yourself when everything is variable and changing.

Many women at this stage feel lost. Like they have lost themselves weighed under the demands of daily life and strife and even under the pressure to be a version of themselves they were before "this stage" or before "it is too late" (fill in the blank). This can feel like an unravelling and the psychological stage at this point is akin to the season of autumn where the trees begin to lose their leaves – to grow stronger for a new flowering eventually in (second) spring or post menopause.

Tracking your cycle is something that will help you immensely in this phase of perimenopause, even when it is going bonkers. Cycle awareness and tracking will give you the power of awareness for yourself firstly but also so you can explain what you are experiencing to those around you and advocate for your needs. You can use a paper or electronic journal or calendar or just write down your overarching symptom(s) every day. You can do this at the end of every day to set up a new habit, maybe stacking it with making your evening cup of tea or writing in your bath or whatever you already do every evening.

Additionally, self-awareness involves you being curious about your stage in life – and leaning into your deeper values as a human. Your values are the lighthouses which keep you heading in the right direction for you, no matter what life throws at you or when. To know your values, you can try remembering a point in your life where everything seemed golden, the golden moments where you wouldn't change a hair on their heads. This isn't just about being "happy" – it is about the moments where you were being present fully with a feeling of "I am exactly where I am supposed to be", "I am at the wheel of the car, even when the car is navigating a wild terrain.

What's important for you about these moments? What were you honouring? What was being honoured?

Then ask yourself or someone who knows you well – what pisses me off? What can't you stand as you make your way through your life? What inspires you on the other hand, in other people, in characters in books or films? You will find a golden thread between all these, these are your values.

Which are your top 3?

The other thing to really know about your values is that they are unique to you because nobody feels them quite like you do. So my version of how "freedom" feels for me is unique to me, my experiences etc. They are also emotional, very emotional, so you may find yourself moved by your own life when you think of them. Bring on the tissues! We need guides and our self-awareness through our inner guidance system is the most authentic guidance we can have. Our values point us in the right direction for us every time.

How do you feel now you have your values like your own private lighthouse?

Stop B: Mindfulness Mountain

Anxiety can be heightened for many reasons at this time. Hormonal, existential, societal, relational, personal, you name it. Have you noticed this?

Mindfulness can rewire your brain, little by little and support your transition and wellbeing moving forward. There have been many studies and there is a large body of research to back mindfulness as a scientifically proven tool to increase our capacity to be with any type of stressor or change period. From reactivity and fear to presence and the power to choose our response. One breath at a time.

The difficult thing about mindfulness is that we are not wired for it. Literally, we are wired for survival, which is why we tend to question and look for the negatives before we appreciate the positives. All of us. Pile hormonal flux and lifestyles that have most women running themselves dry in all this, and you have the perfect storm for depletion, burnout and further exacerbation of stress which flares up any other symptom you could name or imagine.

Let me spell this out for you and stick it on my tour guide's bus: stress gets us more in midlife. It seems unfair doesn't it especially when there is more stress to be had? Ageing parents, teenagers, financial pressures, hormones? Well, yes – and… you can begin to take back your power.

A warning sign is flashing up in front of our tour bus. What might that be? Oh yes I see it now, "It is simple yet it is not easy to be present".

What to do? You are a rebel and you can allow yourself the grace of being present a few minutes each and every day. To just relax your grip, relax your mind, close your eyes and breathe. You don't even have to close your eyes. You can do it whilst you brush your teeth, walk your dog or eat your lunch. Just commit to paying attention fully to the present moment and go from there. Try one breath and then build up daily. When your mind wanders, try again kindly. If that is too hard, you can download an app or a guided practice - there are so many to choose from online.

What is the view like from the top of this mountain, as the clouds part and you are present?

Stop C: Visualisation valley
Visualisation is NOT woo-woo so come on let's visit this beautiful and fertile place of possibility! You know the road we talked about at the beginning ? What did you begin to visualise? We are creating our reality all the time, each moment...but we create our reality based on our past. It's crazy to think, isn't it but our minds work by association. So if you want something to change in your life, you must begin to change something about the way you are thinking. What you are imagining. What you are believing.

These are often called "narratives", stories. We have a network in our brain that serves as the bouncer to the information that is around us and what we allow in and what we don't. You and the people in your past have programmed this bouncer, as have your experiences and beliefs. However, you can change it by giving it new information and thus literally beginning to change your reality.

Begin by imagining what might be, what you want in your future story of you and how you want to feel about it. Go on, what have you got to lose? It is sometimes scary to begin to imagine better, I get it, because "what if" ... but unless you begin to change the information actively, nothing will change. Imagine for example, you love your "holiday" self and want to bring her more to the surface in more areas of your life, more often. What does she do, move like, laugh about, speak like? What kinds of thoughts go through her mind? What is the quality of her feelings? Then get specific, bring her "home" – what is she wearing, moving like, speaking like at work? Is she happy in her job or does she want to ask for a promotion? What job does she do? What house is she living in and with whom? What does she believe about herself? So the filter-bouncer begins to change and you allow yourself new possibilities of being...and can begin to take action accordingly, step by step.

What do you see now that you are inspired to take action on?

Stop D: Self Compassion Sea
Many people believe that they need to be self-critical in order to motivate themselves but in fact they end up feeling anxious, incompetent and depressed. Dr Kirstin Neff's research shows that far from encouraging self indulgence, self-compassion helps us to see ourselves clearly and make necessary changes because we care for ourselves and wish to reach our full

potential and reap the benefits. With self-compassion, her research shows, we lead healthier and more productive lives.

Self-compassion steps in where self-esteem can let us down (e.g. when we fail at something, gain the weight, don't get that job, our relationships are on the rocks etc). The feelings of security and self-worth it provides us with allow us to get up and try again – we become more resilient.

To harness your self-compassion muscle, just notice your inner critic first, and don't allow it to take over, instead just notice it and how it makes you feel. Slowly, you can begin to find ways to talk to yourself like you would a good friend. Every time you flip the script on your inner critic and are kind to you, you build your self-compassion muscle. Watch the landscape change and the clouds part every time you do and see the sun shine on the beautiful sea of self-compassion. This is a beautiful space for self-leadership.

I wonder what becomes possible for you now that you are driven by love for yourself and not fear?

Stop E: Self Expression Shore
Self Expression is vital to communicating your needs and manifesting your unique light in the world. How you choose to live it is entirely up to you – this is YOUR shore, your home.

Living with a sense of meaning and purpose can increase your feelings of self-worth, energise you, give you hope, nurture feelings of being part of something bigger, safeguard from anxiety and depression at all stages in life, buffer you against stress and increase your resilience. Having a sense of purpose can sound lofty and too big to even begin contemplating.

Trust and know that you can start small. What lights you up? What would you not stand by and let pass you by? Reportedly, Naomi Campbell wouldn't get up for under 10k of a morning. What would definitely get you out of bed? This involves intentionality, not living on autopilot in the Groundhog Day effect.

Imagine yourself 20 years from now, who are you becoming when you have been your best and most authentic, lit up self today? And the day after? And so on? Remember that you can make small changes daily and these can lead you in an entirely different direction.

Your Purpose is your North Star – and the amazing thing is… it is already here in you NOW! One lady I worked with recently claimed that cleaning her fridge which she had never done before got the ball rolling, got the spark lit up again and she began to do other things daily that she had told herself were *not her job*, were *too much* (because she was *not worthy*). I wonder what it could be for you? Start small and start today.

Try something new, a new way to express yourself, a dance, a song, that course you always wanted to take, a new hairstyle even.

What is your 70 year old self thanking you for today?

We have reached the final destination in this chapter together. Thank you for letting me guide you. I hope you continue to revisit the different places and gifts of Archipelago of Awareness, Mindfulness Mountain, Visualisation Valley, the Sea of Self Compassion and the Shore of Self-expression and find yourself more supported and with more capacity for being who you are at your core, in midlife and beyond.

Click the QR code to go to my web page of offers for YOU midlife warrior and get started on a journey like you can only imagine is possible in your midlife and beyond...from weekly love notes in your inbox to free downloads and a session just  for you to your 8 week course Embrace, I have you covered with your budget and needs taken care of. What are you waiting for? the music is playing and the lights are on - are you coming to the dance floor?

Journal prompts:

How do you feel now you have your values like your own private lighthouse?

What is the view like from the top of this mountain, as the clouds part and you are present?

What do you see now that you are inspired to take action on?

I wonder what becomes possible for you now that you are driven by love for yourself and not fear?

What is your 70 year old self thanking you for today?

CHAPTER TWENTY FOUR
Discovering New Ways to Make Your Marriage Shine
by Denise Fitzpatrick

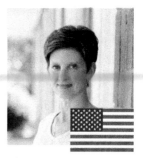

Bio: Denise is a seasoned marriage & relationship coach dedicated to helping midlife women & couples build lasting and fulfilling partnerships. With a passion for helping couples thrive in their relationships, she offers expert guidance and personalized strategies to improve communication, enhance emotional intimacy and strengthen loving connection. Her unwavering commitment to supporting and empowering couples on their journey to lasting happiness has earned her a reputation as a trusted and compassionate advocate for love & marriage.

Business: My Marriage Works
Website: https://www.mymarriageworks.com/

In this chapter we'll explore how changing the way you see your partner and your marriage can bring more happiness into your relationship. What I call a marriage mindset. We'll delve into the power of perception, appreciation, and positive communication techniques that can transform your journey together.

All too often, this critical piece, mindset, gets overlooked or is not even recognized as part of the problem, when trying to make improvements in your marriage. Quite frankly, when we are in a bad place with our marriage all we can think about is how our partner is making us unhappy.

I get it. I once felt that exact way. Thinking it would just be so easy for my husband to do the things I was asking for and we could stop all the unnecessary fighting. My nagging approach to try and get my husband to change was destroying our relationship.

That is until I discovered the power of perspective. Meaning, I began to see how my thoughts and beliefs about my husband were deeply impacting my relationship with him in a negative way. Without even realizing it.

Think of your perspective as a lens through which you see your partner and your marriage. This lens acts like a filter, giving meaning to every interaction, conversation, and moment you share. So while taking different actions, changing certain behaviors is important. Changing the way you think about a problem is even more effective.

For example: If your perspective of your partner is that he is lazy then you will quite easily and readily notice all the examples that prove he is lazy and you will filter out any evidence to the contrary. Your husband may do 5 things to be helpful around the house, he may do thoughtful things for you but when you see him sitting on the couch while you're making dinner and all you can think is "he's so f'n lazy". The tape in your mind starts playing. "I always have to do everything myself, he's so lazy, he never helps out, he's always relaxing while I'm busting my ass".

Notice how you feel when you tell yourself this story. You probably feel angry, resentful and the last thing you want is to be close to him.

The great news is, when you become aware of this internal dialogue and recognize how your thoughts are keeping you stuck in a negative emotional state, you can change this!! When you embrace this idea, you gain control over transforming your relationship. Because, while we can't control other people we CAN control what we do and how we think about things.

Imagine flipping a switch and waking up with a more positive outlook every day. This not only makes your experience smoother but also reduces stress and minimizes frustration. It's a win-win for your emotional well-being.

So how do you have a winning mindset in your marriage?

I created a 3 pronged approach to a healthy marriage mindset that can easily be implemented right away.

1. Partner Perception
The Glass Half Full or Half Empty?
Do you ever catch yourself labeling your partner with

negative descriptions? Like that time they forgot to take out the trash, and suddenly they're the "irresponsible" one. It's as if you have a filter that amplifies negativity.

Trust me, this isn't unique to you. We all tend to view our partners through a negative lens. We're masters at spotting the specks of dirt while missing the rainbow after a storm.

If one or both partners consistently focus on the negatives, what chance does the positive have? It's like looking for evidence to back up a courtroom case instead of seeking the truth. Add in the ubiquitous labels of ALWAYS and NEVER and guess what? Your partner will never be able to show up any differently in your mind. Without even realizing it, you seek evidence to support this narrative and actually dismiss any evidence to the contrary.

I call this the "yeah but" condition. Your partner may have done 5 things right…. Yeah but here's the one thing they didn't do and that's the thing you focus on. It's easy to spot flaws while missing the strengths we fell in love with. When both partners focus on negatives consistently, the positives will struggle to shine through. Your partner will feel stuck in that negative perception forever.

This isn't harmless; it's toxic to your relationship. It fosters resentment, breeds frustration, and weakens emotional connection. The more negatively you paint your partner, the more they'll believe they can never do anything right. It creates a destructive cycle.

Wondering how you can change this?

The first step is awareness. Awareness that this is happening. That you have created negative labels and stories about your partner. Investigate these labels and stories. Are they the truth of who they are? Or is is a part of who they are?

We are all flawed human beings and therefore we all have some less than desirable traits. And also lots of other positive traits. Spend some time remembering what those positive traits are. Remind yourself of these positives each time you find yourself practicing that same old negative story. The key is to have a more balanced perspective. Seeing the positive and the negative. Recognizing that thoughts are not facts.

2. Practice Appreciation: Finding the Silver Lining

Remember that warm, fuzzy feeling when you see a beautiful sunset or smell fresh coffee? That's appreciation at its best. Now, picture weaving this practice into your marriage. It's not just about special dates or gifts; it's about recognizing the good, even in small things. Imagine becoming an expert in your partner's strengths, like a detective uncovering gems in everyday life. And remember, these patterns of thought are habits – and habits can change. When you appreciate and focus on the positives, you nurture a stronger connection. It's like watering a plant; it flourishes.

Appreciation is the fertilizer for your marriage. If you're not nurturing your relationship daily, just like a garden, it will wilt and die. Contrary to popular belief, marriage does not take care of itself after you say "I do".

A practice that is so simple and can easily start right this very moment is to share an appreciation with your partner each day. You can do more than one but start with one as a way to build a new habit. This will also prime you to be on the lookout for things to appreciate. This is a daily task, noticing when things are going well, notice when your partner does something that you could appreciate and say it out loud.

The say-it-out-loud part is very important. I meet with couples all the time who share something they appreciated about their partner. When I ask "does your partner know that", they typically reply, "no". You see, they thought about it, but they didn't share it with their partner. Sharing the appreciation out loud is taking that next step to build a more loving connection with your partner.

After all, who doesn't love to feel appreciated? You are building a more positive energy in the relationship. You are more likely to get more of what you want from your partner when you are doing things to support them changing.

What you appreciate appreciates!

3. Seek Solutions: Navigating Challenges Together
It's hard to move your relationship forward in a positive direction when your tendency is to focus on problems or what's not working. For example: when I'm meeting with clients they want to tell me all the details about what their partner did, said, didn't do, etc. They want to rehash the details of the argument, again reinforcing the problems.

When we stay stuck in problem centric thinking/ focus it's impossible to find solutions. Our brains aren't really even looking for solutions. We just want to feel justified in our complaints.

So I interrupt their story, especially if it's simply airing complaints and criticism of their partner. And I will ask them: "Ok that didn't work for you, that's not what you wanted. What DO you want?"

It often takes people by surprise because they haven't thought about it. They've been so stuck in the problem saturated story/mindset that they haven't considered solutions. Emotions are running the show and it's hard to think clearly.

Recognize when you are spinning in circles restating the same thing, not getting anywhere.
- What am I wanting here?
- What do I want my partner to understand?
- What is important to me in this situation?

Every marriage faces challenges. You know those moments when you feel stuck in a cycle of recurring arguments. Rehashing old fights, minute details of who said what, when and how. Those mind numbing arguments that go round and round with no resolution. Leaving both of you feeling misunderstood, angry and resentful.

This cycle will continue indefinitely, wreaking havoc in your marriage until you shift from focusing on the problem to seeking out solutions.

So how can you start to look for solutions instead of staying stuck in the problem?

Recognize when you are spinning in circles restating the same thing, not getting anywhere.

- What am I wanting here?
- What do I want my partner to understand?
- What is important to me in this situation?

Suddenly, both partners can work together to create change. And communication improves. Instead of playing the blame game, you collaborate, finding common ground.

Rewrite Your Story

In the end, it's all about perspective. You'll always find evidence to support your view, whether positive or negative. So, when in doubt, explore it further. Remember, you have more control over changing your experience than you might realize. You don't need grand gestures; sometimes, a willingness to take the first step is enough.

Let's rewrite the story together. Imagine putting on new glasses that highlight the beautiful moments, shared laughter, and everyday victories. And the exciting part? When your partner sees you making an effort, they will naturally start to shift without realizing it.

Want Simple Solutions to Your
Communication Struggles?
Grab my FREE Guide: The Ultimate
Guide to Less Fighting & More Loving

Notes:

What do I want?

What do I want my partner to understand?

What is important to me in this situation?

CHAPTER TWENTY FIVE
From Diapers to Hot Flashes: Redefining Motherhood in Perimenopause
by Denise Drinkwalter

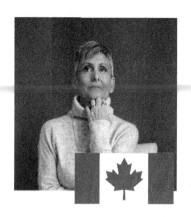

Bio: Denise Drinkwalter is an Empowerment Life Coach who helps women in midlife. Her intuition helps them gain clarity, strength, and perspective. Denise supports moms with grown-up kids, helping them discover new aspects of themselves. Clients praise her kindness and ability to help them release burdens and false beliefs.

Business: Denise Drinkwalter: Empowerment Life Coach for Women in Midlife Years
Website: www.denisedrinkwalter.com

Shifting the focus, mom, from always on them to rediscovering you.

What on earth has unfolded before your eyes? How did you arrive at this juncture? It feels like just a handful of years ago, you were tirelessly shuttling your kids from one event to another, managing an intricate dance of responsibilities, and ensuring your family thrived in terms of nourishment, attire, and emotional equilibrium.

Yet now, your encounters with your kids are fleeting, mere ships crossing in the night, and when you do connect, reality doesn't quite align with your expectations. You once envisioned a future where you and your kids would become the closest of friends as they grew into adulthood. Perhaps you imagined them embarking on global journeys, living in foreign lands, and you longed for the chance to explore these exotic realms through their eyes. Or it could be that you held onto the memory of a time when your children's respect was unwavering, a quality you cherished without realizing until it began to erode.

From diaper changes to the onset of hot flashes and beyond, the question lingers: What exactly has unfolded? How did this chapter of life unravel? And how do you navigate through the whirlwind of intensity, the storm of emotions, the tribulations, and the overwhelming stress? In one instance, you're laughing and carefree, and in the next, you're engulfed in inconsolable tears, the result of an unforeseen shock that's rattled your core, leaving you bewildered and in disarray.

Every one of us undergoes and will undergo our distinct journey through motherhood, yet common threads emerge as we navigate one of the most demanding and simultaneously rewarding roles as mothers, Motherhood in Perimenopause.
The journey of motherhood was never depicted in a way that truly resonated with any of us. As we traversed the formative years of our children, we devised ways to cope, to endure, and

to persevere. Yet as you ponder the trajectory from infancy to late adolescence, how did you manage? What strategies worked surprisingly well for you? Take a moment to reflect and document (jot down in the notes section at the end of this chapter) instances where you witnessed your child take an experience you assisted them through and transform it into a triumph fueled by their dedication and time. How did you support them and in that process, observe their growth?

Did your focus on them lead to your own gradual dissolution over the years of unwavering support? I understand. How did you lose sight of yourself? When can you last remember being unmistakably YOU? Take some time to write down the time when you recall your identity as an individual, detached from the roles of mother, wife, sister-in-law, coworker, and so on. What were your passions? What stirred genuine happiness within you during those times? As you recollect the person you were prior to assuming these roles, what emotions arise? Begin uncovering what genuinely brought you immeasurable joy, embracing your heart, mind, body, and soul.

While entrenched in the role of motherhood, numerous dynamics come into play. One challenge lies in shouldering every burden your children face, often multiple times over. When your children experience pain, you yearn to guide them through the darkness. Sometimes, you step in to solve their challenges alongside them. Yet, intervening prematurely or in an unwanted manner could strain the mother/grown-up child connection. This dilemma arises because you've given, supported, and nurtured your children for 18, 19, 20+ years.

It's complex to shift from that role of constant support to a place where the relationship endures without buckling. Know this: you're not alone in this transition as a mother. It's a voyage we all embark upon, one that can be made less arduous by amassing knowledge and empowering yourself to comprehend that while you'll forever be a mother, your interactions with your adult children can and should evolve to maintain a healthy relationship.

Think back to when you were forging your path to independence when you yearned for and needed your parents' support to succeed on your own terms. How can you now allow your adult children to require you differently while embracing and fostering that change? It involves a shift in perspective and practice!!!

Direct your focus from THEM to YOU! Picture yourself as the epicenter of YOUR universe. As you dedicate time to yourself – by yourself, for yourself, owning of yourself – you not only replenish your own reserves in novel ways but also impart a positive influence on them. You begin to uncover a fresh kind of comfort and happiness, mastering the art of living YOUR life at this moment. This marks the rhythm of existence, an opening to reacquaint yourself with your essence and to grant yourself the time and attention you deserve.

These are the transitions inherent to life's current stage. Jot down one, two, or even three steps you can embark upon for YOU, by YOU, and because of YOU. Venture into exploring the upcoming phase of your Mom journey. Cultivate curiosity about your experiences. Delve deep to learn facets of yourself that might have remained concealed, and observe the transformations that arise from these revelations.

Ask yourself these questions and pen down your responses to unveil more layers of YOU and your identity as an individual:

- What activities ignite my passion? What truly sparks joy in my heart? If it involves aiding others or my children, what specific aspects of those actions bring about happiness?
- What apprehensions do I harbour about growing older? What aspects of redefining motherhood trigger fear, and why?
- How can I immerse myself more in the everyday moments of life? What patterns emerge when I'm stressed, provoked, or emotional in the context of my adult children?
- What responsibilities should I shoulder, and which ones should I release? How can I transition to a stance of accountability in my interactions with my grown-up kids?

Time hurtles from diapers to hot flashes, as we're acutely aware. But are you willing to invest the time needed to uncover the individual you are, and are you prepared to embrace the reshaping of motherhood during perimenopause and beyond because you're empowered to do so? If you're reading this and nodding in agreement, then the answer resounds with a definitive yes. I encourage you to dive into self-understanding, recognize the power latent within you at this life stage, and step back from your adult children's journeys while diving deeper into your own. Take time to immerse yourself in life's moments, embracing the YOU that resides in the depths of your being.

If this chapter deeply connected with you, seize the opportunity! By subscribing to my Newsletter, you'll unlock exclusive weekly content designed to uplift your spirits and help you envision the endless possibilities in  your newfound role as a mother to grown-up kids. While this journey can be challenging, remember that you don't have to navigate the depths of learning all by yourself. Embrace the camaraderie – join our community TODAY!

Journal prompts:

What activities ignite my passion? What truly sparks joy in my heart? If it involves aiding others or my children, what specific aspects of those actions bring about happiness?

What apprehensions do I harbour about growing older? What aspects of redefining motherhood trigger fear, and why?

How can I immerse myself more in the everyday moments of life? What patterns emerge when I'm stressed, provoked, or emotional in the context of my adult children?

What responsibilities should I shoulder, and which ones should I release? How can I transition to a stance of accountability in my interactions with my grown-up kids?

A mothers job is to teach her children to not need her anymore. The hardest part of that job is accepting success.

CHAPTER TWENTY SIX
I Don't Have Time to
Move in Midlife
by Caroline Kerslake

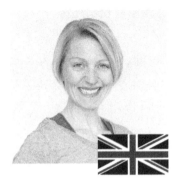

Bio: I work with women on their health and fitness goals, needs, and wants as they enter perimenopause, midlife and beyond. Using movement – through personal training, online exercise class memberships, pelvic floor and core programmes as well as massage and self-care. Because it's not about doing just one thing, it is taking into account your overall wellbeing and understanding that it's all connected.

Business: Complete Fitness and Wellbeing
Website: www.completefit.co.uk

From not having time, to making time. How to get the most out of the time you have for your midlife movement.

Time. Midlife. What a combination. Barely enough time to fit in the day-to-day things that must be done: work, home, kids, parents, appointments, organising, getting from A to B, not forgetting to order this, pick up that, oh and to eat, sleep and relax. We really are in the middle of everything and often find we have more being added to our already full plates.

That may paint a rather overwhelming picture, and maybe one that you may find yourself in. Sometimes something has to give, and it is often what we need more than anything – movement.

As we enter and move through perimenopause, midlife and post menopause, movement becomes a non-negotiable part of our lives that we must pay attention to. Movement for the here and now, but for our future selves too, reducing the risk of age related health issues and conditions.

How are you supposed to find time to move and do the recommended amount of exercise during the week – to work on your cardiovascular system, make sure your bones and muscles are strong as well as taking the time for restorative and relaxing movement?!

The current NHS recommended types and amounts of activity for adults are:

"In general, 75 minutes of vigorous intensity activity a week can give similar health benefits to 150 minutes of moderate intensity activity.
Vigorous intensity activity makes you breathe hard and fast. If you're working at this level, you will not be able to say more than a few words without pausing for breath.
Moderate activity will raise your heart rate, and make you breathe faster and feel warmer. One way to tell if you're working at a

moderate intensity level is if you can still talk, but not sing."[1]

This is great as a guideline, but in real life, just may not be practical. We may not have the time to do 150 or 75 minutes all in one go – or the energy and inclination to either.

So what can we do to get the recommended amount of movement into our day and week, without adding more to our already full plate?

First, let's **look at the time we do have and where it is used.** What does your week look like, break it down to each day, work, commitments, rest time, going out time, etc. Once we can see how our time is being used, we can then see what we have to play with.

And if there are time gaps, block it out, then nothing else can be booked in so you can then plan some movement – or rearrange other things to those time gaps so your day/activities flow better for you.

Then, once you know how much time is available, and knowing where you will be – at home, work, out and about, in between appointments you can look at what you can do in that time. Can you arrange something in this time, or would it be something spontaneous?

What if there are no "time gaps" at all during the week? If you really have trouble finding time then the question is, why is

[1] https://www.nhs.uk/live-well/exercise/exercise-guidelines/physical-activity-guidelines-for-adults-aged-19-to-64/

that – are there things that can be delegated or not done to free up time for you to move?

Then comes the Planning – Like our meals and everyone else's activities we need to plan our movement. If you plan the meals for the week, can you "movement plan", too so you know what you will be doing during the week?

Take a moment to look back on, and look at currently, all you do for your midlife movement. How many classes do you do? What activities do you do? Day to day activities count too, those ones we may not think add up to much.

Then what do you want to do? What type of exercise do you enjoy, have always done, maybe stopped but would love to get back into: walking, running, classes, weights, dancing. If we are limited on time, doing something you do not enjoy isn't worth it. Moving in a way that ticks all the boxes for our midlife health and fitness is important and there are many many ways to do that – each of our preferences are unique to us, just as we are, so we don't have to do "what we should be doing"

- Don't like running, but love to walk, great.
- Not inspired by the gym but like weights, workout at home
- Don't want to be in a group setting but want help and support, use a personal trainer
- Not sure what you want try out, how about some online classes / videos and see what you enjoy.

Rather than doing all the "usual things", take that opportunity for you to do something – what do you feel like doing. Not sure – tune in to how you feel. Do you want to do something quick, fast and powerful, or restorative and gentle?

Having a **movement list** could be helpful. List all the activities you currently do – the workouts, classes, walks etc. Then list the things you may need to do these activities – equipment, location, the time you take for the particular activity needs. Then when you are in a situation when you have more time, or unexpected time you can quickly scan through, pick out what speaks to you and is possible to do and go do it

What about a **habit stack.** You don't have much set time free, or maybe do not want to or able to make the time – we all have times when we "CBA" (can't be arsed). Looking again at your daily activities - work etc what can you do whilst doing something else – we don't want to over multitask but If you are:

- Going into town, can you park further away
- Picking the kids up, get there 5 minutes earlier and walk
- Going for a walk / walk the Dog – add some extra movements in every time you see lamp post/tree e.g. squat, press up
- Having equipment in various places around the house = kettle bell by the kettle, bands on the banister, dumbbells by the door…. Then whenever you are passing you can do xyz.

242

- Waiting for the kettle to boil or while you are cooking, preparing your meal add some movement in.
- Watching a presentation – on a zoom (with the camera off) you could be marching on the spot or stretching
- When it is time to "Netflix" and unwind, change where and how you sit, fidget, stretch, do some movements while you watch.

Focusing on exercise and movement and finding the enjoyment in it - once you start moving, you'll always feel better for doing so, **my top 10 tips and thoughts** on how to do this:

1. Making the time for YOU – blocking it in your diary or taking 5 minutes
2. Getting to know your body and all it can do.
3. Doing something you thought you "couldn't do".
4. Seeing the changes and feeling the changes: physically and mentally
5. Moving your body in a way you never have or haven't for a long time.
6. Reconnecting with yourself, maybe others in a class or a friend during an activity
7. The sense and feeling of "I did it", "I showed up even when I didn't want to" "I put ME first".
8. Taking the steps for your health and wellbeing now and your future self
9. Self-compassion – when things don't go to plan – there is always tomorrow.
10. Anytime is well spent moving – the joy that you did it.

Whatever time you have, 60 seconds a few times a day to 60 minutes 5 times a week, movement is movement and if we are moving, working on ourselves, our strength, mobility, endurance, cardiovascular health, we are on track to ensuring we are doing all we can for ourselves, and that is fantastic.

"5 Moves in 5 Minutes" mini workouts:

Complete Fit "Live" Membership and The "Workout Library" Membership

Moving forward, I will:

1. See when I have time to move – get the diary out and take a look and block out some Me time.

2. Consider how I want to move, what do I enjoy doing or would like to try

3. Think about and implement where can I have items around the house / work etc to help me move

4. Look at my "Why", what do I want to achieve now and for my future self.

"I never regret it when I do it, but I always regret it when I don't"

CHAPTER TWENTY SEVEN
Navigating a
Neurodivergent
Perimenopause
by Kekezza Reece

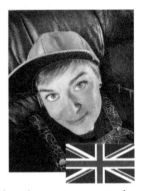

Bio: As an experienced acceptance and adaptation coach, Kekezza Reece's mission is to empower individuals to embrace their unique neurodivergence and find balance in their lives. Through their coaching sessions, they provide a neuro-affirming and trauma-informed environment for their clients to explore their thoughts, feelings, and behaviours. By focusing on self-acceptance and personal growth, they help clients build resilience and develop the skills they need to navigate life's challenges.

Business: KR Coaching and Mentoring
Website: www.krcoaching.co.uk

My perimenopause came before I even knew it was on the horizon. Like countless others, I thought the menopause would be a magic switching off of my monthly cycle. That I would breeze forward without the monthly emotional turmoil or having to carry extra weight in my go-bag. Hopefully, this chapter finds you before yours, and if not I hope it helps you to figure out how to move forward stronger.

There is an increase in women discovering their neurodivergence in perimenopause. I believe this is because of a perfect storm.

Generation X has hit perimenopause, the generation of hyper-independence, the last generation of corporal punishment, and the children of baby boomers. We are an anomaly within the generations, and now we have perimenopause rage. And the internet. Insert maniacal laughing here!!!

More seriously we were the first generation where the boys in our classes were being diagnosed but the girls were not. Asperger's research wasn't translated into English until we were leaving school, and even then it was only used for our male counterparts. It has taken thirty-plus years for the medical profession to realise that there are as many neurodivergent women as there are men. I believe we can thank the actual neurodivergent community for that knowledge.

The advent of social media brought with it a connection the neurodivergent community has never experienced before. I've been an advocate for twenty years, but the changes the internet and social media brought about have been incredible. It has created a neurodivergent friendly communication method which in turn has helped build a vast neurodivergent community. Globally we can now compare notes, collaborate, update current thinking, and advocate in real time. More importantly, we share that knowledge with everyone. There are so many "Actually…" advocates that we can get people's own experience and knowledge, it has meant being able to cut out the academic thinking and disordered language of medical professionals. It means finally understanding what it is like to live with neurodivergence and realise that that has been our experience all along.

I have spent most of my adult life finding ways to cope with an undiagnosed neurodivergent household. The fine line between keeping our heads above water and drowning was carefully managed with whatever strategies I had discovered over the thirty years of trying, failing and learning.

When perimenopause came along my usual coping strategies were no longer working and it didn't take long before a panic set in. Money issues started to form again. Triggers from cPTSD resurfaced. An exhaustion from not knowing what was going on and having to figure it out settled throughout my entire body. Perimenopause is such a massive change to the body's hormonal balance that a lifetime of careful work is undone with the first fluctuation.

Oestrogen is such a powerful hormone, it affects every aspect of your body which is great until it's no longer working in your favour. We have oestrogen receptors in our brain, and along with our neurotransmitters, it helps our brains function. The modern understanding of neurodivergence is that our brains process the world around us differently from some of our peers. This is because of the structure, hormones and neurotransmitters within our brains, and how they work together to help us function. Then perimenopause comes along and upsets that balance. Most women will begin to notice difficulties with the things we've been coping with our entire lives, mood swings, overwhelming emotions, brain fog, sensory responses, or hyper-vigilance, to name a few. We however have a whole other level to deal with as our hormones fluctuate and confuse our body and brain.

I would like to bring your attention to my other chapter as that is relevant now. Go read, simplify, adapt and then come back. Presuming you remember to come back!

1. Camouflaging & Masking

My camouflage partially fell off so unceremoniously that my whole family was shocked. I didn't even know I was wearing one, it was so ingrained from a young age. My every atom was taken up with it and when it fell off my muscles, even ones I never knew were being used, ached for months. I had been holding myself together so tightly for decades that I'm sure it'll take decades to remove the camouflage entirely.

I have learned how to consciously put a mask back on in times of dire need. However, the cost is so high that I have to think about it first. I recognise the privilege of this, as many peri peeps won't have that choice.

If you've never taken off your mask, now is your opportunity. It contributes to the exhaustion and brain fog we experience during this transition, and we all need a safe space where we can take it off and shake off the cost. I started small, in the quiet of my bedroom. I have signs up which tell my family that this is my space and if they come into it they will find me unmasked and freely myself. That if it clashes with their neurodivergent needs, they should leave. I am slowly creating the environment I need, to have the space to unwind, regulate and recharge.

2. Sensory

As I've taken off the camouflage I've explored my sensory needs. I'm using this knowledge to make better accommodations for myself and design an environment that supports my neurodivergence rather than drains it. With perimenopause comes even more attuned senses. My ability to feel changes around me is far more acute, and that comes with the cost of more energy expenditure. Peri has come with some changes that I thought I was imagining and only through talking with other Peri Peeps, was I able to decipher the neurodivergent issues which arise from these changes. I now recommend that all my clients get their sensory profiles as it can help with so many aspects of life from requesting accommodations at work through to setting up a sensory space at home.

- **Auditory (Sound)**

Tinnitus amped up and this has caused additional issues when I already had processing delays. It also means I think I'm hearing things when I'm not, and worse vice versa. I often think I've heard something and there's nothing there. Loop

250

earplugs have helped enormously to aid with sleep (Loop Quiet) and when out and about (Loop Engage). I also use soundscapes when working to reduce the constant hum and beeping in my ears.

- **Visual (Sight)**

Along with tinnitus, I have visual static and this moves around a lot more. As my eyesight deteriorated it also became more visible. I can't tell you how frustrating that is after having paid for laser eye corrective surgery 20 years ago. Combined with the uncomfortable texture and weight of glasses on my face it's another aspect of my sensory experience that I've had to relearn how to cope with. I take regular breaks from my spectacles and also pay for the Transitions filter and varifocals, so once they're on my face I don't have to keep changing them. Otherwise, every time I had to change them it reset my comfort level and it would take ages for my face to get used to them again.

I have also developed floaters in my left eye which are incredibly distracting and can cause temporary fuzziness in my left eye. The optician claims I will learn to ignore them, but I think they are underestimating the combined power of Autism and ADHD. I constantly see them, and then get distracted by them. I have yet to find a solution for this, although I do know you can get them removed if the floaters are bad. As I have enough scar tissue on my eyes I have chosen not to do this. We'll see how long that lasts if they get worse.

- **Olfactory (Smell)**

I have dreaded this section because my journey with smells has always been a difficult one. My gag reflex is easily tripped and it can take hours for the nausea to settle back down again. Yes, with peri this can get worse. From a more attuned nose to the changes within our bodies this is the worst aspect for me.

Body odour changes have left me reeling at times, they remind me of boys' locker rooms. The overwhelming nature has led me to buy a diffuser for my bedroom so I can, at least in my room, create a calming olfactory environment. I have also started buying extra large wet wipes so I can wash every morning, something my dynamic disabilities don't always allow for.

Period Blood changes its smell. There I said it. I'm so over Taboos! It reminds me of the bag of beef mince I can discover at the bottom of my fridge that I've forgotten about. You know what I'm talking about, don't deny it! The lingering smell in the bathroom doesn't help much either. I did go through a period (pun intended) of using nappy sacks to hold the pads and pons so the smell was less, but then I discovered menstrual cups and I haven't looked back.

- **Gustatory (Taste)**

I am a gustatory stimmer. Between humming so my mouth and nose vibrate through to using certain flavours and textures to help regulate. This also changed with perimenopause, when my IBS flared and I had to cut certain foods out of my diet, spicy foods being a notable absence. I have had to search around for alternatives and I am still searching for a low FODMAP chewing gum, if anyone knows of one?

- **Tactile (Touch)**

This brings me to the tactile nature of peri periods. I had to move to a cup after many years of tampon and pad use because I started cramping more. I hit the point of being rolled up on my bed crying into my pillow. Someone suggested the menstrual cup could help with cramping and I figured it was worth the change. I found a cup with a valve that empties straight into the toilet because I am not always able to empty and refit a cup due to being a wheelchair user. My cramps have lessened to such a degree it is now rare for me to need my hot water bottle. I also stock disposable gloves so I do not have to touch them with my bare skin, something I have always struggled with.

Reusable pads are so much more comfortable for me as well, I rinse them under the cold tap and throw them straight into a laundry bag. The entire thing goes into the wash. I wish these had been around when I hit puberty, being an adult while going through these changes is an advantage.

I have also gained weight as my metabolism has changed, along with managing moderate to severe Myalgic Encephalomyelitis. This has meant I have changed my wardrobe. I can not tolerate the feeling of a tight waistband and have moved, almost exclusively, to dungarees. I now dopamine-dress, and it has brought so much joy into my every day. A subject for another day.

- **Vestibular, Proprioception and Interoception**

I am only at the start of my journey into this aspect of my sensory world, and it is already such an eye-opener. I have Alexithymia. It affects my ability to pick up my body's messages such as hunger or thirst. It doesn't affect my emotions though, although that is not the case for everyone.

Essentially it meant that as a teenager I could forget to eat until I got dizzy, and it was only because my vision changed that I realised that I had forgotten to eat. I have set a reminder for so long that I forget I eat to an alarm. When I became a neurodivergent life coach I did so much self-exploration that I am now ultra-aware of the changes I have made over my adulthood to function. That being said I am still reconnecting to my body due to camouflaging for so long.

I have learned that these aspects of my sensory profile are as important as the 5 senses most people are aware of. I try to think back to a time before I camouflaged and hid my needs from those around me. My vestibular and proprioception needs are under-reactive and I will always seek out new experiences, it's why I love theme parks..... at least in term time and on weekdays. I miss being whirled around on a swing by a twisted up chain, flying through the air on a Witch's Hat, or climbing trees and dangling from the branches. I used to have a hammock and I would spend hours reading on it in all manner of positions. I look forward to being able to afford one in my garden once again. I keep eyeing up those internal slings that you can fix to the ceiling and hope to experience them.

3. Communication

My neurodivergent perimenopause brought with it extremely uncomfortable anxiety and returning panic attacks. I sat in one for months before I found a way to lessen it. During this time I found my ability to recall words started to falter. Some days, due to the power of also having Myalgic Encephalomyelitis, I can have difficulty speaking at all. From slurring which makes me sound drunk to knowing what to say but being unable to form the words with my mouth. There are several jokes floating around our household about cucumber curry, the delightful (note sarcasm here) experience of the first letter being correct but the word being totally incorrect. I don't even know I'm doing it until I keep getting confused faces looking back at me.

I became aware of Augmented and Alternative Communication several years ago when my son developed situational mutism. Although he doesn't use AAC, it didn't take long before I installed Proloquo4Text on my iPhone. Even if I do not use it all the time, it relieves the stress of talking which usually means I can talk. As someone who was called a chatterbox the irony of losing my voice at times is not lost on me.

4. Summary

This is my experience, I share it to give you a peek inside a neurodivergent perimenopause. I hope you find it reassuring that it can get better. I know we are so much more than masks, sensory profiles, communication issues and executive functions, but I am hoping this gives you somewhere to start when navigating the chaos of a neurodivergent perimenopause.

My biggest takeaway from this chapter is GET TO KNOW YOU. Your greatest weapon is knowledge. Get to know how YOUR neurodivergence affects YOU. It's a classic *"You don't know what you don't know until you know."*

Scan the QR code to find out more about neurodivergence in perimenopause

Notes:

CHAPTER TWENTY EIGHT
The Chaos of a
Neurodivergent
Perimenopause
by Kekezza Reece

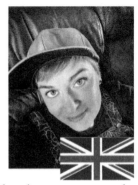

Bio: As an experienced acceptance and adaptation coach, Kekezza Reece's mission is to empower individuals to embrace their unique neurodivergence and find balance in their lives. Through their coaching sessions, they provide a neuro-affirming and trauma-informed environment for their clients to explore their thoughts, feelings, and behaviours. By focusing on self-acceptance and personal growth, they help clients build resilience and develop the skills they need to navigate life's challenges.

Business: KR Coaching and Mentoring
Website: www.krcoaching.co.uk

The first thing I need you to know is it gets better. Hopefully, you haven't already hit burnout and this is the closest you're going to get to it.

Even if you're not (knowingly) neurodivergent, I implore you to read this chapter.

Perimenopause brings so many changes to our bodies that it can feel like our life is descending into chaos. When you're Neurodivergent the balance between coping and not coping is so carefully managed that if you didn't know perimenopause was coming your way, or you don't know that you are neurodivergent, life can become so unmanageable so quickly. And it feels like it came out of nowhere.

If you already know you're neurodivergent, this is the time to get to know how it affects you and the coping strategies that you've already found, a lot of them subconsciously, need to be understood to be able to simplify, hack and strengthen them.

If you don't know you're neurodivergent, but you're reading this chapter, something tells me that in the back of your mind, you've suspected that you're wired differently, highly sensitive, or have always wondered how others seem to sail through their adulting. Or this is the first time in your life you've hit a wall and you don't know how to get back to the person you were before.

1. BASICS

The absolute back-to-basics is Nourish, Hydrate, and Nurture. Nourish is about making sure you're eating to fuel your body with what it needs, filling it with the good stuff. It also means everything in moderation including moderation. Nourishing your soul means sometimes you need that blowout because life is about living. Hydrate so your brain can function, we're made of water and it needs replenishing.

Finally, nurture means sleeping enough, being gentle with yourself and spending time doing things which bring you pleasure and joy. It means getting to know you, the person you've become through your life so far, and what you need to feel nurtured.

Now you've got your foundation sorted we can move on to changing things up.

2. SIMPLIFY

When your perimenopause has swept you off your feet, look at everything you dropped when you hit the floor. *You don't have to pick it all back up again.* Now is the time to look at your life and prioritise. You get to create the life YOU want and make the changes to make it happen. If you need to write out everything you do to be able to sort through it, do it. Go get that pen and paper and list it all out. EVERYTHING. I used an entire stack of Post-it notes, stuck them on my wall and rearranged them over a few weeks until I had an order of importance. **Then I binned the bottom third.**

Sounds so easy but those weeks were painful whilst I moved notes around and designed what I wanted and needed in my life. We've added and collected responsibilities over the last twenty or so years and it's time to have a good clear out.

3. HACK

I must admit, this is my favourite part. There are so many

ways we can adjust how we do things, this is when you get to experiment.

Environment

I always start with your environment because it can make such a difference in how you do things. Move things to where you'll get visual reminders.

Can't find your keys? Put a hook by your front door to hang them on as soon as you walk in the door.

Put a reminder up on your mirror in the bathroom so when you're brushing your teeth every morning you can have a glance up and see what YOU are asking you to do next. I put vinyl stickers on mine. They remind me to do my face cream before I brush my teeth. And "Only Light and Love" to be mindful of others, but mostly of myself. Trust me I'm the least airy fairy a person can get, but we all need reminders to be gentle with ourselves.

Create a designated space for your sensory needs, it doesn't have to be an entire room. Find a space or time when you won't be disturbed, and set it up to provide the sensory feedback your body is craving. Once created, this space will give you the comfort and time-out your body needs to cope with all the chaos going on around you, and within you. Mine is a "Joy Box", it's a shoebox filled with bits and pieces I have found that meet my sensory needs, I pull it out when I need that time out.

Technology

Use it!!! If you think you're going to remember the bits you need in the supermarket, you're not! This is not a failure.

There's nothing morally wrong with using tools to support you in day-to-day life. You are expecting your brain to do everything it did in your twenties, plus all the jobs and responsibilities you've picked up over the last 20+ years, plus everyone else's, whilst it's coping with the fluctuation of a key component it needs to function. Stop it.

Most of us carry a smartphone, if this doesn't work for you you're going to need something more than a notebook. You need audible, tactile and/or visual reminders, something that makes you stop in your tracks and take notice.

There are so many apps available it's about finding what works for you, and your cycle, and I'm not talking about your menstrual cycle. I'm talking about your neurodivergent one. Mine sits between 6 weeks and 6 months, depending on how busy I am. My whiteboard lasts 6 weeks before I don't see it anymore. I can make it last longer by using different coloured pens, getting someone else to update it each month, and having more than one board. The Tiimo App lasts 6 months, then I have to move to Owaves App for a bit, then the Google Suite, before I cycle back around to Tiimo.

Your neurodivergent cycle is essential to work out, mainly so you can stop beating yourself up when things suddenly stop working. Remember the "Only Light and Love" sticker? This is why.

The list of how much I've scooped out of my brain and use tech to do is so long, reminders, notifications, a smartwatch which buzzes every hour, different sounds for different reminders, yes even the Red Alert Klaxon from Star Trek features in my lineup.

Using tools to help us is not cheating, it's working smart. Quite frankly even if it was cheating here's your permission to do so. Everyone's strengths are different, remembering to buy toilet rolls just isn't yours. Use the tools available to help you. Offload your brain, and give it some much-needed rest from juggling everything.

4. STRENGTHEN

Here's where I talk about executive functions (EF). So what are executive functions?

They're your brain's ability to interact, connect and process the world around us. Most of the tasks we do as adults use them, and most people's EF develop and strengthen during their childhood and teenage years. If you're neurodivergent your mixed bag is, well, divergent. It needed to be before society changed so radically over the last couple of hundred years. Now we're stuck with a mixed bag of functions in a world not designed to use them.

Thankfully our brains retain the ability to grow and change, this is where you do that. But ONLY if you've managed to simplify and to hack.

Trying to strengthen your executive functions whilst still doing ALL of the adulting is like swimming, fully clothed, with added weights and against the current. Why would you?

Get an overview of your executive functions and pick a middle ground one, start small, and, I can feel my ADHD screaming, repetition strengthens. When you get bored with that one, pick another one. *Remember your ND cycle.*

It's like learning a new language, small spurts, repeated every day, strengthen them. 5 minutes at a time. Reward yourself when you succeed, don't beat yourself up when you don't remember. Go back to technology and set yourself reminders.

5. REBOOT

Use this chance to focus on yourself and what you need to move forward again. Once you've sorted your basics, simplified, hacked and started to strengthen, you'll be able to consider where you want to take the next chapter of your life. Many of us reach this point and feel like we've been on a conveyor belt. We went through educational systems, got jobs, built families whether that's partners, children or friends, got promotions, got caught up and pulled along, but haven't had a chance to stop and look at how far we've come, how much we've achieved or whether we are where we wanted to be. Now is our reboot.

Scan the QR code to find out more about
neurodivergence in perimenopause

Notes:

CHAPTER TWENTY NINE
Not on HRT? All is Not Lost...
Here's How You Can Support
Yourself
by Geraldine Joaquim

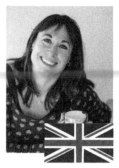

Bio: Before training as a hypnotherapist, I worked in international marketing. Unfortunately I found myself 'running on empty', which manifested in being high functioning but not really engaged, particularly with my growing family – there was just no spare capacity to do anything outside the routine and that's not much fun! I needed a change... So, in 2016 at the age of 46 I started training to become a Solution Focused Hypnotherapist.

Since then, I've helped numerous clients with a diverse range of issues, but I have found a particular interest in sleep disorders, women's health and menopause, and healthy weight loss.

In 2020 I was diagnosed with breast cancer which prompted me to explore non-HRT solutions to help support my own perimenopause symptoms, so I've been there/done that!

Business: Geraldine Joaquim
Website: www.geraldinejoaquim.co.uk

Whether it's due to your medical history, family health risk, or you just want to navigate this life stage in your own way, it can seem like HRT is touted as the only solution.

Everyone else is on the HRT party bus, but you didn't get an invite!

Then there's the higher risk of developing osteoporosis, dementia, heart disease... it can be anxiety-inducing, loading more stress on top of whatever you're already struggling with.

But don't despair! Maintaining your good health through perimenopause is not all about taking a tablet, smearing on a cream, or slapping on a patch!

There are ways you can support yourself – and even if you are on HRT it's worth doing these too because feeling good is a combination of your thoughts and actions. When you take control of your health, you're also boosting your confidence in yourself and your own abilities without waiting for others to 'fix' you.

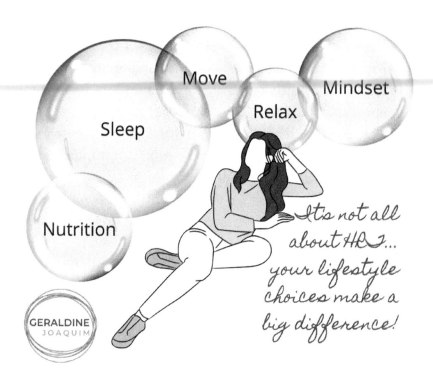

It's not all about HRT... your lifestyle choices make a big difference!

Sleep

Sleep is the foundation of your good health, everything else is impacted by it. And let's face it, you know what it feels like when you haven't had enough sleep. Brain fog, feeling hyper-sensitive, mood swings, exhaustion, and you probably find yourself reaching for convenience foods to shore up flagging energy levels which leads to weight gain... sound familiar? Not to mention health consequences like high blood pressure, heart disease, or neuro-degenerative diseases such as Alzheimer's (one study suggests sleep deprivation could increase your dementia risk by 20%).

So, what can you do about it?

- **Prioritise your sleep** – make it important, create a bedtime routine that prepares your mind and body for sleep.
- **Make your bedroom a haven for sleep** – comfortable bed and pillows, a cool and dark room, minimum noise, remove all entertainment and electronics.
- **Alleviate physical issues as best you can** – night-time trips to the loo could be down to drinking/eating late so allow 90 minutes before going to bed to switch off your digestive system. Or you could have inflammation in your body: help to remove excess fluid by going for a short walk before bedtime or lying on your back with your legs elevated for 15-20 minutes. For aches/pains, think about managing them with pain killers or topical creams, or gentle massage which could form part of your bedtime routine (you might want to speak to your doctor about specific pain treatment options). If you suffer from hot flushes then have props available (a fan, fresh night clothes, pillow to swap out a soggy one).
- **Address stress** - if you're struggling to get to sleep, or wide awake in the middle of the night, it's time to address your stress levels. Sleep is an important brain processing time but when you have too much going on your brain struggles and wakes you up (seeing a therapist may be a good option).
- **And if you can't sleep?** If you've been struggling to sleep for 20 minutes, go into another room. Do something relaxing like listening to music or reading (keep lighting

low), that isn't too stimulating, and when you feel sleepy go back to bed. If you still can't sleep, do it again... and again. It may take time for your sleep pattern to re-establish but you are training your brain to recognise that being in bed means going to sleep, not being awake!

Nourish

Looking after your diet is about eating sensibly and choosing good quality fresh whole foods over ultra-processed convenience ones. Think of it in terms of "does this food support my good health or hurt it?" And as for the link between food and menopause, studies have shown that eating a Mediterranean-style diet can help. It's rich in foods that contain phytoestrogens (natural oestrogens from plants).

Eat lots of these: vegetables, fruits, nuts, seeds, pulses, whole grains, fish/seafood, olive oil
Eat these in moderation: poultry, eggs, dairy, wholegrain bread
Eat rarely: red meat
And avoid these: refined sugar, refined grains, refined oils, processed meat, highly processed foods

And you can support progesterone levels with foods containing vitamins C, E and B6, zinc, magnesium.

It's also a good idea to moderate your alcohol consumption as it's a central nervous system depressant. It does have sedative qualities so whilst it might seem like it relaxes and helps you to sleep, it raises your body temperature which interrupts your sleep.

Whether you're on HRT or not, being very overweight or obese has many more serious implications than a fluctuation in your hormones. It's linked to a number of chronic health conditions including heart disease and thirteen types of cancer, as well as impacting on cognitive and emotional functions like memory and mood.

Move

One of the consequences of getting older is an increased risk of developing osteoporosis, and that's one of HRT's benefits: "It (HRT) can help to prevent osteoporosis in the years around the menopause" (Royal Osteoporosis Society).

Up to the mid-30's our bodies are in an anabolic state which means that it's easy to build and maintain muscle. As we age, we move into a catabolic state which involves the process of breaking down tissue so we have to work harder to maintain muscle - not to mention counteracting the effects that gravity has had on our bodies!

As well as eating foods high in calcium and getting plenty of vitamin D, including strength training that builds strong muscle and supports your bones will help stave off age-related decline. This doesn't have to mean hours in a gym lifting weights (although it can if you enjoy it!), use your own body weight with activities such as yoga or Pilates. Do what you enjoy doing and you'll soon feel the difference.

Relax

Being on the go all the time is like keeping your foot on the gas pedal, revving your 'engine' so you end up running on adrenaline and cortisol.

Cortisol production literally steals from your dwindling progesterone and oestrogen supplies which upsets the already fragile balance.

As your ovaries stop producing progesterone the adrenal glands take over, which is also where cortisol is made. Your body prioritises cortisol breaking down any available progesterone in the process. And oestrogen is produced in balance to cortisol: the more cortisol you make, the less oestrogen, and vice versa.

So, a key part of balancing your hormones is relaxing. It can be active or still, it can involve getting your creative juices flowing or watching Love Island(!), whatever works for you as long as it allows your mind some space to free-flow and you enjoy it.

Another important component here is the production of serotonin, your mood stabilising hormone, it helps to cap the release of cortisol.

To create a steady flow of serotonin:

- **Purpose**, having a sense that you are part of something bigger than 'I', recognising your value and contribution.

- **Interactions** with others, feeling connected.
- **Thoughts**, taking control of your attention, acknowledging the good stuff, recognising when your thoughts are spiralling into negativity (and having strategies to move them on).
- **Actions**, movement and exercise, hobbies and doing things you enjoy, lifestyle choices.

Mindset

We are predisposed to see things negatively, but this just amplifies what's wrong which increases misery, fuels anxiety, makes you feel bad – which increases cortisol levels! Your brain tries to give you what it thinks you want – if you focus on the negatives, you'll get more of them.

It's an important skill to be able to step back and reframe what's happening.

- **Retrain your brain** to recognise the good stuff, instead of dwelling on the negatives – ask yourself what's been good about my day? Start with one thing and gradually build to two, three or more. Acknowledge that there are some good things in your life, no matter how bad things might seem!
- **Accept what's happening now**, and it's not forever – change can feel frightening, which increases your stress levels and produces more cortisol. Acceptance can bring some relief in the moment and keeping in mind that this is a period of change, it's not permanent.

- **Focus on what you want,** not what you don't want – if you focus on feeling helpless or in pain, you'll get more of the same! Instead ask yourself what you want, what will make you feel better, and seek solutions which will help you cope (and you'll release serotonin which will help too!)
- **You can't help how you feel** but you can influence it – it can seem like all these emotions are happening to you, and whilst it's true to a degree you can move them on through changing your thoughts, behaviours and environment. If you're sitting on the sofa feeling miserable, it's time to get up and go outside for a walk (or make a cup of tea, or clear out a cupboard, whatever small task you can manage), start to consciously move those thoughts on, change what you're doing, and where you are.

These are some quick tips and if you need help managing your stress levels or coping with symptoms of menopause, help is available – the biggest step is asking.

Stop struggling on your own, help is at hand. Contact me now for a free no-obligation chat. Quote 'perihub book' for 10% discount off your first session. It's time to get back to the real you.

275

Notes:

What one thing will you take away from this chapter?

What difference will it make in your life?

Now make a commitment to yourself, write your action out on a post-it note and stick it somewhere you'll see every day as a reminder: On xx day, I will do xx activity.

CHAPTER THIRTY
What happened to my libido?
Where are my orgasms?
by Naomi Harris

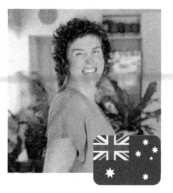

Bio: Naomi is a sexual pleasure and genital pain specialist. She supports women to heal their pelvic and sexual numbness, lack of libido and orgasm, pain and discomfort, so that they can live a turned on life full of pleasure, passion and epic sex.

Business: The Pleasure Naturopath
Website: www.thepleasurenaturopath.com

Female sexuality and desire is complicated, and the challenging thing is that perimenopause can only make it more complicated.

I am a member of lots of different online groups that support women as they enter this time of their lives, and one of the most common questions that is asked in these groups is about what can be done with the changes to libido, desire and body responsiveness that seems to happen for so many women.

'What can I do? I used to love having sex, but now I just want to throw something at my partner when he even looks at me'

'What can I do? My head wants to have sex, but my body is dry, and it just hurts.'

'What can I do? I don't come any more, and when I do it is small and disappointing and I feel frustrated afterwards.'

The comments for these questions are always filled with advice: different techniques or toys to try, different locations to spice things up, or things to read or watch or listen to or fantasise about. And while a lot of the suggestions might be valid, they are missing the most important thing when it comes to female sexuality, arousal, and turn on. What is missing is the understanding that it is SO complex! There just isn't one solution that is going to work for all, or even for most.

Every woman's body is so different, and the reasons that you are experiencing what you are is unique to you, which means that trying out all of the suggestions might actually lead to more shut down in the long term (more about that to come). And the suggestions, while they might make orgasm more accessible, or turn on more possible, are missing something else.

With female sexuality, we have to think about more than just the body parts involved. If we no longer get physically aroused, or orgasm is harder to come by, or our vulva or vagina is dry or hurting, we tend to focus on the body part that isn't cooperating, and try to work out what we can do about it directly. Whether there is a cream that will help. Or a patch, or an implant or a tablet.

But as women, we are so much more than just the body part that isn't behaving. When we think about our genitals and our sexuality, we also need to think about what is impacting us emotionally. And mentally. We have to consider what we believe about sex as we get older and also our sexual and sensual history.

Then there is what we really want and need. Or whether we feel safe, or have shame and fear. How much patience and trust we are receiving from ourselves and the people that we are with. What our energy levels are like. All of our unspoken histories, irritations, anger, frustration and resentment that we hold to the ones that we are trying to relax and get sexy with. Just how long our to-do lists are, and how much energy they leave us with at the end of the day. And so much more.

So, let's talk for a minute about how to not make things worse, before we move on to how to make things better. What can actually make things worse is buying a vibrator or the latest toy or some kind of cream or device, and trying out the 'just keep pushing until something happens' approach to arousal.

There are a number of reasons this can make things worse.

The first is because not slowing down enough to listen to your body and actually learn what is needed can lead to more numbness, turn off and disconnect. None of us like being pushed around and told what to do. Your clitoris and genitals are no different!

If your body is not getting aroused, and you try to push it towards arousal like that is the thing that absolutely has to happen right now, and your body has been telling you that it isn't interested in arousal right now, thank you very much, one way that your body might deal with this is by shutting down even more.

The other thing is that if you are already experiencing numbness, or turn off, or dryness, or even pain and discomfort, there is a reason that your body is giving you these symptoms. And when you just push towards orgasm, you are ignoring what it is that your body is trying to communicate with you, and a body that doesn't trust that it is being listened to isn't one that is going to relax and open into wetness, and pleasure and orgasm.

Another reason to think about, is that as women, we are taught to have sex like men, and quite simply, your body might be one of those that is not interested in that dynamic anymore.

Sex for many men is quite straightforward. There is an action that is being taken, and a goal that is being moved towards, it's like getting a job done, a fun, feelgood job that is!

For many of us women, the truth about sex is that it is more like a swim in the ocean with goggles and a snorkel. First we want to float over here and take a look around. And then maybe slowly flipper over there, and see what there is to see. And then put some more effort into it and swim down deep and find something beautiful, and then surface and take in the sunlight on the water, before we go back under for some more exploration. And we can do that for hours.

So many of us might be tired of sex that is focussed on an end result, and might feel like there has to be more, even if we don't know what it is. And that can also lead to shut down, and turn off, because on a subconscious level, we are ready for more.

And lastly, you might just be really, really tired. Really, really, *really* tired.

Tired of your energy being pulled in so many different directions. Tired of all of the ways that everyone is leaning on you and demanding things of you. Tired of all of the plates that you have spinning in the air, and how nothing ever seems to get any easier.

Just tired.

And a tired body, one that doesn't get enough positive attention from you or from your partners or lovers, is one that might just not have enough juice in the tank to find its arousal and wetness. Being that tired isn't a good basis for feeling sexy.

So, what can you do about it?

Here is the thing. We are taught that our pleasure and orgasm come from other people. 'He gave me an orgasm'. 'She turned me on'. 'He made me cum.' 'They showed me what my body could do.' With the changes in our bodies, we are so often waiting for the cure or the fix to come from outside of ourselves. From our lovers, or our toys, or our doctors. Or we are looking to make something happen, in a body that might not have enough juice in the tank for that to happen.

So, the first thing that we need to do is to slow down, and really pay attention to our bodies.

I know, it's not easy. But like anything good, it's worth it.
The great thing is that slowing down and paying attention to your body, and waking up that sleeping beauty part of yourself, can be the most rewarding, and most fun homework you will ever do.

Which leads me to my top 5 tips for turning on your turn on and pleasure:

1. Time and attention keeps your body alive and juicy.
Stop putting pleasure at the bottom of your to-do list. And yes, I know that we are all way too busy and life is too crazy and giving more time to pleasure is the last thing you want.

So, make it manageable. When you put lotion on your body, slow down and notice what you are touching. Touch your vulva, even if it is just for a few moments every day. Taste food that goes into your mouth. Look at beautiful things. Smell scents that light you up. Use your senses so that it becomes part of your everyday life.

2. Go slow. Really slow.

Boring I know, but the payoff is worth it. Slow down! We are taught that sex is fast and rough and you have to get to the finishing line. What if you slowed down and enjoyed the journey more, yes, even with just yourself? Explore your body as if it was something completely new to you. Find out what really lights you up and turns you on, and take the time it needs for that to happen. How do you know that you don't get aroused or feel the way that you used to, if you don't go slow enough, or take the time it takes to find out?

3. Learn how to breathe.

If you really want to feel more in your body, you need to learn how to breathe properly. Your breath is the most powerful tool that you have to relax your tension, grow your pleasure, to move it around your body, to have those kinds of orgasms that you have only heard about but never experienced. Learn to breathe into your belly and your pelvis so that you can really feel.

4. Touch yourself like you are someone that you love.

This is so important! If you can touch yourself like someone you love, you bring your heart into the experience. And the more your heart can be part of your lovemaking, yes, even just with yourself, the richer and deeper and more powerful your pleasure will be.

5. Stop trying to make something happen (aka enjoy the journey, don't focus on the destination!)

So often we go into pleasure with an eye on the end result. No sex or self pleasure without orgasm. And then the whole focus of the experience becomes the orgasm. But what if you changed the focus to how much you can feel right now, in this moment, and then orgasm just becomes a bonus?

And always remember: your pleasure, your orgasm, your wetness, your lust and desire and turn on... they are YOURS.

And,

If you have ever felt like you were less of a woman because you couldn't find your arousal no matter what tricks and toys you tried, then hear this!

You are not broken!
You are not less than!
You are not undesirable!
You are not worthless!
You are not wrong!

Your worth isn't decided by how much your body responds.
Your lovability isn't decided by your libido.
You are so much more than that.

AND! If your turn on and libido have become an issue in your mind that you can't let go of. If the feelings of shame, or guilt, or longing are with you all the time.

Or if you just want to take a stand for yourself.

That you are worthy, and loveable, and desirable, and you want your sex life to be an epic part of your life,then healing is also available to you.

Your body can be awake, and aroused, and alive, if that is what you are dreaming of.

If you want to find out what is really possible for your pleasure, desire, libido and orgasm, and what you can do to get there, download my free Pleasure:Amplified guide for more support.

Notes:

CHAPTER THIRTY ONE
Pelvic Health in Perimenopause:
A Physiotherapy Perspective
by Nicola Travlos MCSP HCPC
BSc (Hons) Physiotherapy

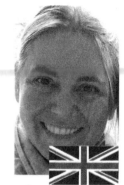

Bio: I am passionate about Pelvic Health and specialise in integrated Pelvic health for women in the Peri and Menopause. I provide a safe space to understand your pelvic health concerns, guide your treatment options through education and discussion and facilitate healthful living to optimise your pelvic health and wellbeing. We work towards you living an active life in a pelvic safe way based on your individual needs.

Business: Invictus Pelvic Health
Website: www.invictuspelvichealth.com

Embrace the changes of peri and menopause as a journey towards strength, resilience, and self-discovery. Your body is a masterpiece in progress, and pelvic physiotherapy is your toolkit for maintaining vitality and well-being.

The Menopause transition can significantly affect the health our pelvic organs (the bladder bowel and uterus) the pelvic

287

floor muscles, and other tissues such as connective tissues or fascia ligaments and tendons. This can lead to symptoms such as bladder and bowel dysfunction, pelvic organ prolapse and general vulvovaginal symptoms. The great news is that pelvic symptoms can be managed with the specialist help of Pelvic Physiotherapy, together with a team approach including your GP and Urogynaecology nurse or consultant and menopause practitioners, as well as taking a look at pillars of your overall health and wellbeing and the lifestyle changes that can be made.

What exactly can Pelvic Physio do?

Pelvic Physios undertake an assessment to talk to you about your symptoms and get a picture of when they started and how long you've had them for. It takes about an hour and will likely include a check of your posture, your breathing and may include an external and internal examination of the vulva and vagina and rectum if needed. We check the appearance of the tissues, look for any dryness or skin changes as well as an assessment of your pelvic floor and muscles to see if you are doing pelvic floor exercises correctly and can help to guide you as to whether you need to go to see your GP and/or get a referral to a consultant for further investigations if you have any concerning symptoms.

I am using the correct terminology with hopefully a simple explanation so if you are needing to describe your symptoms to a doctor or other health professional you can use the right terminology.

What bladder symptoms might you experience in perimenopause?

- **Urinary Frequency** - Going to the toilet more often.
- **Urinary Urgency** - Getting a strong overwhelming urge to pee, this is when the actual bladder and the muscle in the wall of the bladder contracts involuntarily.
- **Urinary Urgency Incontinence** - You can't control urinary urgency,you may leak before you get to the loo.
- **Stress Urinary Incontinence** - Leakage of any amount of urine with movement or activity which increases the pressure of the abdomen on the bladder such as coughing, sneezing, laughing or leakage during any movement activity such as walking, running or jumping.
- **Mixed incontinence** - When you get a mixture of stress urinary incontinence and urgency incontinence.

How to help your bladder

Have you been checked for a bladder infection? If not, head to the GP to rule that out with a mid stream urine (MSU) and then move on to the rest of this advice.

Are you drinking enough of the right type of fluid?

Typically we would encourage you to drink 1.5 to 2l per day of water, squash or decaf tea or coffee and herbal teas. We would encourage you to avoid drinks such as tea, coffee, alcohol, fizzy and diet drinks that contain irritants such as caffeine and aspartame.

STOP JICing - Try not to go to the loo Just In Case (JIC).

Do some Bladder Training [1]. If you are having recurrent urinary tract infections or having persistent pelvic pain after a UTI, please contact your health professional and get referred to a Bladder Hero to help you as you need specialist care.

For stress urinary incontinence (SUI) getting good at contracting AND relaxing the pelvic floor can be helpful and in fact this is the first line of treatment recommended in the NICE guidelines, also using the KNACK which is a pelvic floor contraction[2] **before** you cough or sneeze has been proven to help with SUI.

What kind of Bowel Symptoms might you experience in the perimenopause?

- **Frequency** - Going for a bowel movement more often.
- **Urgency** - Feeling a strong urge to go for a bowel movement.
- **Bowel incontinence** - Experiencing symptoms of bowel incontinence can range from smearing of your underwear, having difficulty wiping clean after a bowel movement as well as being unable to control the loss of any amount of poo or wind from the back passage.
- **Constipation** - Straining to empty the bowels.

There are 2 types of constipation:

[1] https://www.yourpelvicfloor.org/media/Bladder_Training_RV1-1.pdf
[2] https://docs.google.com/document/d/1l1DnO-xSmRWUZv1Th8MBIOZ3s1zv4dyg-8F-brCvn-s/edit?usp=drive_link

290

- **slow transit constipation** where the poo takes a long time to get around the system and is therefore dry and dehydrated when it comes out.
- **obstructive defaecation** – this is when the poo is difficult to pass no matter what the consistency and can be related to prolapse, too much straining and an overactive and dysnergic (uncoordinated) pelvic floor.

Looking at your bowel function and managing constipation

Physios are brilliant at giving bowel advice and we generally encourage you to mimic a squat position on the toilet by putting your feet on a stool. We also ask you to breathe your way to pooing by starting with diaphragmatic breathing to open your ribs and relax your pelvic floor and your abdomen. Allowing your tummy muscles to relax and bulge out encourages the sphincter and pelvic floor muscles to relax and open. We can help you to coordinate your muscles if you are struggling with obstructive defaecation. You can also try saying sounds which can help the pelvic floor to relax such as MMMOOOO.

Listen to your call to go for a poo, don't ignore it.

We take a look at what you are eating and encourage you to add healthy non processed foods into your diet, as well as different types of fibre (soluble and insoluble) to optimise your stool consistency to make it easy to pass. Aim to drink 1.5 to 2l of fluid per day, and a daily walk or movement of at least 20 mins can get the bowels moving.

If you have more complex issues such as IBS (irritable bowel syndrome, IBD (inflammatory bowel disease), neurological issues, blood or mucous in your poo or have food intolerances or allergies we may encourage you to get a referral to a dietician or a nutritionist for specialist help or to return to your GP to ascertain whether you need laxatives or rectal irrigation and or further investigations from a gastrointestinal or colorectal specialist.

What is a prolapse?

Pelvic Organ Prolapse (POP) is the movement of the pelvic organs, the bladder, bowel or uterus from their supported position in the pelvis and symptoms are often felt as a heaviness or dragging sensation in the pelvis, feeling or seeing a lump in the vagina and the changes in bowel and bladder habits you may be experiencing could be related to this.

There are different types of prolapse but the main ones you may experience are:

- **A cystocoele or front wall prolapse** is a movement of the bladder from its usual position and creates a bulge or bulging sensation through the front wall of the vagina.
- **Rectocoele or back wall prolapse** is a change in the position of the bowel tissues which causes a bulge or sensation of a lump on the back wall of the vagina into the vaginal canal.

- A **uterine prolapse** is movement of the uterus into thevaginal cavity from its usual position.

How can Physio help POP?

We help you with posture, assessing your pelvic floor so that we can understand whether it needs uptraining (strengthening) or downtraining (relaxing) or both. We help you with learning how to breathe and how to contract and relax your pelvic floor as well as teaching you how to manually release your scar tissue and managing intra abdominal pressure through managing constipation, lifting well and can train you in hypopressive exercise (if qualified). This is a breathing technique adapted from yoga which can be helpful for management. We can also examine you in standing and give you advice on where to go to be fitted with a pessary if needed. We do a thorough examination of your pelvic floor and can give you the correct advice on when and how to do pelvic floor exercises and how to integrate this into your exercise programme safely and into your activities of daily living.

What kind of vulvovaginal (outside/inside) symptoms might you experience in Peri?

- **Vaginal atrophy** is when changes in the tissues of the vulva and vagina leads to thinning of the tissues, shortening and tightening of the vaginal canal.
- **Vaginal dryness** - Often women talk about a feeling of dryness in and around the vulva and vaginal area.

293

- **Dyspareunia** is the general term for painful intercourse.
- **Genitourinary symptoms of menopause** is the term encompassing all the above effects including urinary frequency, urinary infection, dryness, itching, pain sensations and general inflammation.

How can physio help?

Hormone fluctuations and changes in muscle tone can contribute to pelvic pain or discomfort and Pelvic Physiotherapy can provide guidance on maintaining vaginal health through the use of non hormonal lubrication, through exercise and manual therapy and other techniques such as biofeedback, vaginal dilators and release work. Pelvic floor physiotherapy may involve breathing, relaxation and stretches to alleviate muscle tension and reduce pain.

Childbirth Injuries and the perimenopause

You may have experienced an injury during childbirth such as:
- **a second degree tear** of the perineal muscles between the vagina and the anus.
- **3rd or 4th degree tear** of the perineal muscles and extending into the tissues of the external (3rd deg) and internal anal sphincter (4th deg).
- **episiotomy** – a cut from a scalpel into the perineum which helps the baby to be born vaginally.
- **an assisted delivery** with use of forceps or ventouse during birth.

- C section this can be planned or emergency and createsscar tissue which can be helped by physio treatment.
- **Divarication or diastasis recti** – this is a tummy gap in the muscles and fascia experienced after pregnancy which does not always resolve. If you are concerned please see your GP or physio or exercise specialist who can assess you and help you with a rehabilitation plan.

You may not experience any ongoing symptoms from a childbirth injury until the perimenopause when the hormone changes start to affect the tissues of the pelvic floor and you may start to experience urinary and bowel symptoms, prolapse or pain symptoms so it can be really helpful to have postnatal check up from a pelvic floor physio post birth. It's never too late postnatal to have a check up!!!

Impact of Lifestyle Factors on Pelvic Health

Remember to take note of lifestyle factors such as the quality of your sleep, stress management, diet and fluid intake, and exercise as this all has an impact on your pelvic health.

What exercise can we do safely in Peri?

It is important to note that unless you have an underlying medical condition it is generally safe to do physical activity in peri and menopause and you can build up to a weekly exercise regime that works for you as an individual depending on your health and wellbeing.

Exercising can be highly beneficial for overall health such as bone density, mental health and cardiovascular health as well as managing some of the associated symptoms of peri.

Breathing well and good posture are essential baselines for exercise. This is because our breathing muscle, the diaphragm, has a synergistic movement with the pelvic floor. This reflex action can be disrupted by stress, lung issues, constipation, pregnancy and childbirth so if you are not breathing well, it is important to re-educate breathing. Breathing also helps to stimulate the vagus nerve which sends messages of rest and digest to your nervous system and digestive system and encourages the pelvic floor to release and relax.

We need strength, balance and dynamic flexibility through our bodies and this helps with posture, supports our pelvic floor and thus our pelvic organs. Examples of types of exercise that encompass all of this are yoga, Pilates, Tai Chi, Barre, walking, swimming, weight training and cycling. Pelvic physios or Women's Health Specialist exercise trainers such as Holistic Core Restore (R) Instructors can provide personalised guidance based on your specific needs and any underlying health conditions.

Have a look at my blog on what to expect from seeing a pelvic floor physio.

Notes:

Please use this space to write down any of your pelvic symptoms and how often you feel symptoms daily/ weekly/monthly.

Try pelvic floor exercises – do you feel you are doing them correctly and are they helping your symptoms? If not seek help from a Pelvic Physio.

Are you aware of any other issues that may affect your pelvic floor such as breathing, posture, foot mobility, previous injuries or surgery?

Take your notes page with you to your physio, GP, consultant or other health professional to help you navigate your joint decision making.

CHAPTER THIRTY TWO
Creating Your Peri Plan
by Kathy Fritz

Bio: Kathy Fritz is a board-certified master hormone coach who coaches women in perimenopause and menopause to get rid of the weight gain, hot flashes, and sleep & hormonal issues so they can feel like themselves again, regain their energy, and lead a longer, healthier life. Her clients lose weight, rediscover their energy, feel sexy, and stop thinking they're losing their minds. Kathy's background in education gives her the expertise to individualize material so her clients can go from where they are to where they want to be.

Business: Kathy Fritz Coaching
Website: https://kathyfritzcoaching.com/

The essential first step before you go diving into new habits is to ask yourself: What stage of change am I in?

You've learned from some unbelievable experts in this book, and you're ready to tackle this perimenopause thing.

So you should just jump into it, right? Not exactly.

Too often, I see women get excited about the food, movement, and lifestyle shifts they could make, try to make a bunch at once, and only last a week with all of these new habits.

Or, they feel overwhelmed with all of the information and aren't sure where to begin. So they don't begin.

You don't have to follow either of those paths!

Having a clear Peri Plan will increase the likelihood that you'll make changes and stick to them.

In this chapter, I'll give you some information about habit change, explain how to approach perimenopause so you get the results you want, and give you a few templates to support you.

Step 1: Create your 3-Month Vision

Here's the thing about habit change- if you try to do it without a clear vision of why you're doing it, you're bound to give up.

So before you even decide what change you'll make first, I want you to imagine 3 months from now.

Grab a piece of paper and jot down the answers to these questions. Write this in the present tense and in the affirmative (what you want, not what you don't want). Go a little crazy-be detailed, descriptive, and have fun with it!

- What do you want for yourself by the time 3 months have passed?
- What would you like more of in your life?
- What elements of your health and wellbeing do you want to improve?
- What values come through in your vision?
- What motivates you to achieve it?

Now take a look at that vision of health, that vision of wellness, that vision of life as you want it and know in your bones that it is possible.

Client example:

In 3 months, I make choices that serve me almost without thinking about it because I am in a state of freedom. My habits give me this freedom, and I have successfully reprogrammed my day-to-day schedule so that my choices easily flow. I know which food and movement choices are best for my body, and I choose them 90% of the time. I handle my stress effectively, and this helps me sleep better. I feel content and confident. I am committed to having a high quality of life that I can share with my husband and children.

Step 2: Break Down Your Vision

Now that you have this beautiful overarching vision of what you want to achieve, what do you need to get there? Take a moment and brainstorm everything you can think of that you want to change so you can reach your 3-month vision. Don't let limiting beliefs hinder you. Just go crazy and list anything and everything that comes to mind.

Now, I know it's tempting to get right to it (or maybe not to start because there's a lot on that paper!), but before you start any new habits, you've got to complete Step 3!

Client example:

Food	Movement	Lifestyle
- Cut out processed foods - Figure out food sensitivities - Learn how to eat for my body now - Stop eating chocolate every day - Stop snacking	- Stop sitting at my desk all day - Walk more - Do yoga or lift weights - HIIT training - Move more throughout the day	- Sleep through the night - Feel less stress - Find time for myself - Feel more gratitude and peace - Spend more time with my husband

Step 3: Figure Out What Stage of Change You're In

If changing our habits was easy, then I wouldn't have a job.

The fact is, without support, it's incredibly challenging to make changes that are lasting and sustainable.

There are a lot of reasons for this (and diving into those is beyond the scope of this chapter), but the main reason is women don't pause to ask themselves which Stage of Change they're in. They just pick a category and start trying to make a whole lotta change in that area. Or they pick one new habit in multiple areas.

But the essential first step before you go diving into new habits is to ask yourself: What stage of change am I in?

This is actually a complex question because your stage of change is not the same for all areas of your life.

You could be in Precontemplation when it comes to taking a dairy break, but you're in Preparation for adding strength training to your weekly movement routine.

To figure out your stages of change, let's geek out for a moment: there are six Stages of Change according to the Transtheoretical Model of Behavioral Change.

For this chapter's purposes, I'm going to introduce you to the first four.

Name	Definition	What it means for you
Precontemplation	You *do not intend* to take action for the next 6 months.	You're *not ready to change* a habit, even if you want to change it.
Contemplation	You *intend* to take action sometime in the next *6 months*.	You're getting ready to change a habit, but you are having doubts and delaying taking action.
Preparation	You intend to take action within the next month.	You're *ready to change a habit*, but you are also feeling some fear, likely of failure.
Action	Congrats! You're *making changes* to impact a habit!	You're *doing the work* while feeling loads of emotions—joy, excitement, discomfort, and more! This is the most demanding stage.

So whatever you're looking to change or add first, make sure you're in Preparation. If you're not, there's work to be done before attempting any change.

You can try journaling or vlogging to better understand why you're not in Preparation around a particular habit or category. Ask yourself:

- Do I want to make a change in this area?
- If I don't intend to take action within the month, what is holding me back?
- What support can I get to help me work through these barriers?
- What would it take for me to want to take action within a month?
- What are the pros of changing? What are the cons of changing?
- How would it feel to change? How would it feel to stay the same?
- What information would help me be more likely to change?

If moving through these questions by yourself feels daunting, then look into getting a board-certified coach.

We help our clients move to Action around habits they want to change and stay accountable to themselves when they're in Action.

Client Example:

Things I want to change (from Step 2)	Stage of Change	Priority
Sleep through the night	☐ Precontemplation ☐ Contemplation ☑ Preparation	☑ Week 1 ☐ Week 2 ☐ Week 3+
Feel less stress	☐ Precontemplation ☐ Contemplation ☑ Preparation	☑ Week 1 ☐ Week 2 ☐ Week 3+
Find time for myself	☐ Precontemplation ☑ Contemplation ☐ Preparation	☐ Week 1 ☑ Week 2 ☐ Week 3+
Feel more gratitude and peace in my life	☐ Precontemplation ☑ Contemplation ☐ Preparation	☐ Week 1 ☑ Week 2 ☐ Week 3+
Spend more time with my husband	☐ Precontemplation ☑ Contemplation ☐ Preparation	☐ Week 1 ☐ Week 2 ☑ Week 3+

Client Story

When we started working together, Tina shared that she relied on constant coffee consumption to get through her day, so she had no interest in taking a coffee break. Since she was in Precontemplation, we started in a different area where she was in Preparation.

Since improving her sleep was part of what she wanted, I asked her if she was interested in better understanding how caffeine impacts a midlife woman's body. She said yes, so I sent her some information.

After reading through the information and asking some questions in our session, Tina decided she was ready to try a coffee break. She didn't cut it all out at once though, as she didn't want to experience severe caffeine withdrawal.

She created a new caffeine reduction goal each week until she fully swapped out her full caf coffee for decaf, which she enjoyed in the morning.

Tina maintained this routine for three weeks, and her sleep steadily improved until she was regularly sleeping deeply for 8 hours a night.

Tina gradually moved from Precontemplation to Action by:
- Gathering information
- Asking a knowledgeable professional her questions
- Approaching her body from a place of curiosity

- Connecting her decision to try decreasing her caffeine to her big goal of sleeping better

If Tina had forced herself to take a coffee break when she was still in Precontemplation or Contemplation, she likely would have given up early in the experience.

But by waiting until she was invested and curious, Tina was successful and able to make a decision that was best for her body.

OK, now you're ready to take a look at your list from Step 2 and have an honest conversation with yourself.

As you look at your list of brainstormed ideas, which ones are you in the Preparation Stage for?

Step 4: Begin Your Baby Steps

Look at the ideas you've marked as "Preparation," then pick the one you believe will be easiest for you. Habit change is all about early wins!

Does this idea need to be broken down into smaller steps? It probably does!

Take that change you want to make, and break it down into 3-4 gradual steps that are specific, measurable, achievable, realistic, and time-bound.

Client example:

Big goal/desire: Sleep through the night.

Baby steps:
- Turn off all lights by 10:00 5 out of 7 days.
- Do all bed prep by 9:30 5 out of 7 days.
- Read a light, easy fiction book from 9:30-10:00 5 out of 7 days.
- Finish streaming shows by 8:00 5 out of 7 days.

As you look at each goal you've created, ask yourself:

On a scale of 1-10, how confident are you that you can do this? If you're below a 7, what can you do to change that? How will you stay accountable to this goal?

Again, if attempting this process feels overwhelming, find a board-certified coach who specializes in perimenopause.

You do not have to go it alone!

Moving Forwards

As you continue to work towards having the perimenopause experience you want, remember:
- Modest goals work best.
  - Cutting out all gluten might be ideal, but is by no means modest. Maybe not eating gluten when you are home is a more modest, achievable goal.

- Break a larger goal into concrete, small goals.
  - To cut back on gluten, you could replace traditional pasta with chickpea pasta, spaghetti squash, and sweet potato noodles.
- To form new habits:
  - Cue- change the cue response from a bad to good habit. For example, after a challenging day at work (the cue), instead of drinking a few glasses of wine (the old cue response), treat yourself to your favorite salad, roll on your favorite oil, and take a 30-minute walk with your rock out music (new cue response).
  - Keystone habits- find the habits that when you change or keep up with them, everything else seems easier (these habits give positive ripple effects). Commit to these habits, and when you have a slide, return to these habits first.
  - Act as if- believe you can do it, that you can change and sustain change

As you make changes to your food, movement, and lifestyle habits, you will have successes and slides.

Just keep going!

And remember, you are not alone, you do not need to suffer, and you are worthy of your 3-month vision!

Whether you are in Preparation and would like support as you enter Action, or you're in Precontemplation and have no idea how to get to Action, Kathy can help!

Check out her website kathyfritzcoaching.com or scan the QR code to join her Facebook group and get access to weekly free trainings on all things perimenopause!

Journal prompts

3-Month Vision (from Step 1):

Things I want to change (from Step 2)	Stage of Change	Priority
	☐ Precontemplation ☐ Contemplation ☐ Preparation	☐ Week 1 ☐ Week 2 ☐ Week 3+
	☐ Precontemplation ☐ Contemplation ☐ Preparation	☐ Week 1 ☐ Week 2 ☐ Week 3+
	☐ Precontemplation ☐ Contemplation ☐ Preparation	☐ Week 1 ☐ Week 2 ☐ Week 3+
	☐ Precontemplation ☐ Contemplation ☐ Preparation	☐ Week 1 ☐ Week 2 ☐ Week 3+
	☐ Precontemplation ☐ Contemplation ☐ Preparation	☐ Week 1 ☐ Week 2 ☐ Week 3+

Baby Steps (from Step 4):

Big goal/desire (from row in above table where you are in Preparation):

Baby steps that are specific, measurable, achievable, realistic, and time-bound.

1.

2.

3.

And remember, you are not alone, you do not need to suffer, and you are worthy of your 3-month vision!

CHAPTER THIRTY THREE
Why is Everyone
Pissing Me Off?
by Julie Blatherwick

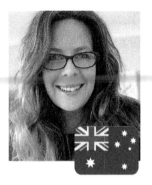

Bio: Julie Blatherwick is an educator and coach who supports women in remaking their life after an abusive relationship. Trauma can take time to emerge; abused women can remain unaware of how what they've experienced continues to impact them – sometimes for years. Perimenopause and the associated hormonal changes can, in some situations, trigger the emergence of trauma.

Business: Remaking Your Life
Website: Remakingyourlife.com

As our hormones change, many of us experience changes in our emotional life including feeling frustrated or annoyed at those around us. Don't dismiss what these emotions are about – they could actually hold the key to what you want and need in your life and in your relationships.

As our hormones change, many of us experience changes in our emotional life including feeling frustrated or annoyed at those around us. This annoyance, frustration or irritation could be aimed towards your significant other, your children, other family members or work colleagues. It might even be a frustration at life in general, a wanting of something different, a wanting of something more, or perhaps it is just those socks that you are sick and tired of picking up off the damn floor. All of this is really common and normal. But what is also really common is that many of us say things like, 'these things shouldn't bother me' or 'it's not really a big deal'. We gaslight ourselves into believing that what we are feeling, or the size of our feelings, is not OK so we try to ignore them, minimise them, or wish them away. There is a lot of messaging out there that tells us that women are emotional, too emotional, because of our hormones so is it any wonder we gaslight ourselves about what we are feeling; we're already coming from the viewpoint that we shouldn't be making a big deal of things or that things shouldn't bother us in the first place. The problem with denying our emotions is that they tend to build and build until we explode at someone; and then we add another layer of guilt on top of everything else.

Our hormonal fluctuations and changes don't necessarily create emotions but rather can make them more intense or bring into focus feelings we didn't consciously know we felt. If you are having a hard time managing your emotions then yes, talk to your doctor or OBGYN for sure, but maybe also use this time to check in with yourself. The hormonal changes you're experiencing may have turned your emotional world upside down, and you might need help with managing those emotions so you are better able to cope, but don't dismiss what the emotions are about – they could actually hold the key to what you want and need in your life and in your relationships. These changes can make it more difficult to pretend to ourselves and to others around us that everything is OK. Perhaps what you're feeling is new or perhaps it has been hidden under everything else, perhaps it's something that you've never had a chance, or taken the chance, to look at and examine. Be curious, investigate yourself, take some time to reflect on what is actually at the core of the changes in your emotional world you might be facing.

Give yourself permission to be unhappy, unfulfilled, disgruntled, to want more or to want different for yourself, if that is what you are feeling. Those feelings are understandable for a lot of us, because we have been fed so much bullshit about what it is to be a woman – no wonder so many of us feel the way we feel! Think about the messaging we regularly receive starting in childhood and continuing today (although slowly changing!). Women are seen as the nurturers, the caregivers, the homemakers yet many of us work outside of the home as well. Statistically we do the majority of the chores at home. Yes some will say that the chores are split 50/50 but there are a few problems with that claim: it's often not really 50/50; chores commonly assigned to women are usually done daily, every day, relentlessly day after day, whereas 'men's' chores are often done weekly, monthly, ad hoc, or can more easily be outsourced; women carry the mental load of knowing and organising what needs to be done and when, letting others know what needs to be done and when, and checking that things have not only been done, but done correctly. On top of all this we, the women who we've been led to believe are 'too emotional', also carry the emotional load of our relationships, the checking in, the starting of difficult conversations, the helping others to contain their emotions, the emotional load of child rearing, the conflict resolution. If you have been doing this for everyone else for a few years or a few decades, is it any wonder that you've had enough or are frustrated at the very least?

Not only have we been taught that this is our lot in life, but we're also taught that wanting to do all of this is part of what it means to be a woman. It can be challenging to step outside of that and ask if that is really true for us. And it is completely and utterly OK if it is true for you, if it does make you happy. But how do you know unless you actually stop and have a look at it? Challenge yourself on what you believe, disentangle yourself from the traditional gender roles we have been taught to live by. If you end up wanting or believing the same, that's great but make sure it is you and not the bullshit we've been taught to think over the years from our parents, from the way society was when we were growing up, from the media, from the patriarchy. Start putting yourself in the front and centre of your life and see what you want and what you need.

Disentangling yourself from these messages so that you can put yourself front and centre of your own life is easier said than done. We have been subtly told that everyone else's needs come before ours – we do the opposite of what is recommended in an airplane when the oxygen masks drop down. And everything that we've been told about what it means to be a woman, a good woman, and what a good and successful life looks like, has influenced what we believe is important to us, it's influenced our values. Our values, the things we hold most important, influence our decisions, the choices we make and the behaviour we display. When we live a life aligned to what is important to us then we tend to be happier and more fulfilled. When we live a life that isn't aligned properly or completely with our values then we can experience angst, frustration, disillusionment, irritability.

During this stage in our life, it can be pertinent to re-evaluate what is important to us because our values can change as we reach different phases of our life. Or maybe we've been ignoring our true values because they didn't align to what we've been told 'should' be important to us and we are at a point where we can't ignore that anymore. Either way, this period of our life can be a great time to define what our values are now.

Taking time out to reflect and reevaluate what is actually important to us, the real us, the us that is disentangled from the messaging we've received about what 'should' be important to us as women, can take us to the bottom line of why all of a sudden everyone is pissing us off. Reflect on what is important to you when it comes to your relationship with your significant other, your home life, your family, work, or whichever area of your life is giving you the shits.

Defining your values, defining what is important to you, then gives you a compass; values become something to help guide your decisions, your choices as well as your boundaries. And the more specific the better. For example, people refer to 'family values' but what does that really mean? Different families might prioritise different things. Different members within one family might prioritise different values, which is where things can come undone if they're not defined and communicated. So, start with yourself and try to define what your top 3 values are for a part of your life that is pissing you off. Ideally values should be action based so you're looking for words or short phrases that include verbs or adverbs. And they should be you-focused rather than others-focused; this is about what you need or want in a particular area of your life.

For example, a few years ago now, I realised that I wanted to live 'more peacefully'. This became a core value for many areas in my life, not just one. I started looking at what in my life moved me further away from peace and what areas moved me closer to peace. I started making decisions based on what will bring me closer to peace in the longer term, what will give me a little more peace right now? I can't live a life with no stress because unfortunately that is often a part of modern life, however, I can prioritise minimising the impact it has on me. This change in focus impacted my relationships, my boundaries and my self-care.

Having a clear definition of your values has a strong link to your boundaries and your self-care. Living aligned to clearly defined values based on what is important to you, and not what we've been fed from the patriarchal society we live in, allows you to live in a way that honours you and that is self-care, that is self-love. It also allows you to set boundaries more clearly and firmly because you are more confident about them. You don't need to justify your boundary, you don't need to apologise for it, or gaslight yourself out of it because it is based on what is important to you, on what you want and need in a given situation or relationship.

Allow yourself to be pissed off at the people who are pissing you off. Don't disregard it or make yourself wrong. Look at why it is pissing you off and how perhaps traditional gender roles or gender-conditioning is influencing either the annoyance or the guilt you might feel about being annoyed in the first place. Disentangle yourself from all the messaging you've received about how things should be and focus on what is actually important to you. Define those values clearly and start living aligned to those values in a more conscious way. And if this means changing or adjusting the boundaries you have with those around you, do so confidently, and kindly, knowing that you have just as much right as anyone else to honour what it is that you want and need.

If you would like some defining-values inspiration, download my free comprehensive Values List to help get you started! And, as always, please reach out if you'd like some additional support along the way.

Journal prompts:

My top 3 values are …

What these values mean to me is …

To live more aligned to my values I need …

Living aligned to clearly defined values based on what is important to you, and not what we've been fed from the patriarchal society we live in, allows you to live in a way that honours you.

CHAPTER THIRTY FOUR
Harnessing the Power of Breathwork for Perimenopause
by Polly Warren

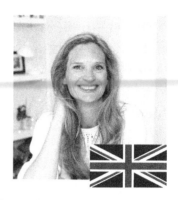

Bio: Polly is a Perimenopause Health and Wellbeing Coach, ex primary School teacher, mum of 3 and host of The Positive Perimenopause Podcast.

Polly believes no woman need suffer during their menopause transition and understands that many simply lack the support, knowledge and wellness tools they need to thrive in what can often be a transformational time in a woman's life.

Using her extensive menopause and wellness knowledge along with her wide range of coaching skills, Polly supports women to thrive through perimenopause and beyond through 1 to 1 coaching and group programmes.

Business: Polly Warren Coaching
Website: www.pollywarren.com
Instagram: @pollywarrencoaching

Welcome to the wonderful world of breathwork—a powerful tool that can empower you during your perimenopause journey.

Why Does Breathwork Matter?

It's no secret that most of us struggle with the everyday pressures of life. We're living in an age where we're busier than ever and because most of us are disconnected from our bodies, it's easy for us to become buried in feelings and emotions that we don't know how to deal with or process. For many of us, the norm is being constantly stressed, anxious, worried and overwhelmed. Breathwork is like a reset button. It allows us to be still, be with ourselves and breathe and feel through our experiences.

We were given the tool of breath since birth, but most of us are unaware of how powerful and transformational the breath can be. By tapping into the healing power of the breath, we can enhance our well-being, promote emotional balance and cultivate resilience during perimenopause.

The Science Behind Breathwork

Breathwork isn't just some woo-woo practice; it's rooted in science. The way we breathe can actually influence our body and mind in profound ways. It's like a bridge connecting our conscious and unconscious minds, and it even talks to our autonomic nervous system.

When we breathe consciously, we can activate the parasympathetic nervous system, which helps us to relax and reduces stress. Plus, breathwork influences hormone regulation, oxygenates our cells and even strengthens the mind-body connection. All of this together makes breathwork a secret weapon for managing perimenopause and keeping those emotions in check.

The Benefits Of Breathwork

Breathwork offers a myriad of benefits that supports us during perimenopause. Some of the most common benefits are:

· **Instant Stress Reduction and Anxiety Relief**
Breathwork's immediate effect is the easing of stress and anxiety, it's like a sigh of relief! When we practise conscious breathwork, we activate the parasympathetic nervous system and trigger the relaxation response. This state of relaxation helps to counteract the effects of chronic stress, which can disrupt hormonal balance. As stress hormones decrease, the body can recalibrate itself, allowing for a smoother transition through perimenopause.

· **Sweet Dreams and Cool Nights**
Breathwork can play a vital role in promoting hormonal balance. It promotes better sleep quality and helps in managing common perimenopausal symptoms like hot flushes and night sweats. Because breathwork promotes better oxygenation and circulation, it can have a positive impact on the endocrine system, facilitating the secretion and regulation

of hormones.

· Giving Your Organs A Boost
Oxygen is like fuel for your body's engine. With each breath, you're sending a fresh supply of oxygen to every cell. This oxygen fuels the metabolic processes necessary for cell growth, repair and maintenance. By engaging in intentional breathwork, the amount of oxygen delivered to our organs is enhanced, which allows them to operate optimally and efficiently.

· Bye-Bye Toxins
Our body needs a detox every now and then and breathwork helps with that too. More oxygen means your body can clear out waste more efficiently, leaving us feeling refreshed and revitalised.

· Get Energised
Breathwork invigorates every part of our being as it enhances oxygen utilisation and mitochondrial activity. Mitochondria are the powerhouse of cells, responsible for generating energy through processes like oxidative phosphorylation. By supplying an abundance of oxygen to your cells through breathwork, we promote efficient energy production, leading to increased energy and vitality.

· Mental Clarity Boost
Oxygen is a brain booster, helping you think sharp and stay focused. Oxygen plays a crucial role in brain function, acting as a catalyst for neurotransmitter synthesis and maintaining

neuronal health. By enriching our bloodstream with oxygen-rich breaths, we provide our brain with the essential resources it requires for optimal cognitive performance.

· **Emotional Liberation**

Perimenopause can be a bit of an emotional rollercoaster! Breathwork gives you a safe space to connect with and process emotions. It's a bit like an emotional detox, providing a healthy way to release pent-up feelings and emotions.

· **Letting Go of Lingering Trauma**

Life experiences, including past traumas, can leave energetic imprints in our bodies, affecting physical and emotional well-being. Perimenopause might bring some of those to the surface, but breathwork helps to release them. Through deep and conscious breathing, it's possible to tap into the body's wisdom, allowing it to express and release stored emotions and tensions. In the presence of a skilled breathwork facilitator, you can experience profound healing journeys, unburdening yourself from emotional weight you may have carried for years.

· **Trusting Your Inner Wisdom**

Perimenopause is a time of transition, prompting many of us to re-evaluate our lives and priorities. Breathwork can be instrumental in connecting with our higher self, inner wisdom and intuition. As the mind quiets down during breathwork practices, the channel to access higher guidance opens up. Through consistent breathwork practice, we can gain clarity about our life's purpose, desires and direction. This newfound connection with our inner wisdom can lead to empowered decision-making and a deeper sense of self-awareness.

Breathwork Techniques To Try

Practical breathwork techniques provide tangible tools for incorporating the power of the breath into your daily life. The following techniques can be tailored to suit your individual preferences and needs and are easy to do by yourself, allowing you to harness the transformative potential of breathwork during perimenopause.

Diaphragmatic Breathing

Diaphragmatic breathing, also known as belly breathing or deep breathing, is a foundational breathwork technique that focuses on engaging the diaphragm muscle to promote relaxation and activate the parasympathetic nervous system. This technique can be done in a comfortable seated or lying down position.

How to Practise:
- Find a quiet and comfortable space to sit or lie down.
- Place one hand on your chest and the other on your abdomen.
- Inhale deeply through your nose, allowing your abdomen to expand as you fill your lungs with air. You should feel your lower hand rise while your upper hand stays relatively still.
- Exhale slowly and completely through your mouth,

feeling your abdomen gently contract.
- Continue this deep, rhythmic breathing, focusing on the expansion and contraction of your abdomen.
- As you breathe, you can imagine inhaling positive energy or calming colours and exhaling stress or tension.

Alternate Nostril Breathing

Alternate nostril breathing, also called Nadi Shodhana or Anulom Vilom, is a technique that balances the flow of energy between the two brain hemispheres. It is believed to support hormonal balance and enhance mental clarity.

How to Practise:
- Sit comfortably with a straight spine.
- Close your right nostril with your right thumb and inhale deeply through your left nostril.
- Close your left nostril with your right ring finger, release your right nostril, and exhale through your right nostril.
- Inhale deeply through your right nostril.
- Close your right nostril, release your left nostril, and exhale through your left nostril.
- This completes one cycle. Repeat for several rounds, focusing on your breath and maintaining a steady rhythm.

Box Breathing

Box breathing, also known as four-square breathing, is a imple technique that helps promote calmness, focus and balanced nervous system activity.

How to Practise:
- Sit or lie down in a comfortable position.
- Inhale deeply through your nose for a count of four.
- Hold your breath for a count of four.
- Exhale slowly and completely through your mouth for a count of four.
- Pause and hold your breath for another count of four.
- Repeat this cycle for several rounds, gradually increasing the count if comfortable.

Guided Imagery and Visualisation

Guided imagery and visualisation combine breathwork with the power of your imagination to induce relaxation and reduce tension.

How to Practise:
- Find a quiet and peaceful environment to sit or lie down.
- Close your eyes and take a few deep, relaxing breaths.
- As you continue to breathe deeply, imagine a serene and calming scene, such as a beach, forest or meadow.
- Engage your senses in this visualisation. Imagine the sights, sounds, smells, and textures of your chosen scene.
- Sync your breath with your visualisation. Inhale as you immerse yourself in the positive imagery, and exhale as you release any stress or tension.
- Stay in this visualisation for a few minutes, gradually bringing your awareness back to the present when you're ready.

Remember, the key to effective breathwork is regular practice. There's no one-size-fits-all approach so experiment with these techniques and find the ones that resonate with you the most.

If you're seeking deeper experiences, consider exploring breathwork sessions with a trained facilitator, either online or locally, to guide you through more advanced practices, often to music which takes you on a journey and helps you navigate powerful releases in your body.

Keep in mind, your perimenopause journey is uniquely yours. So be kind to yourself as you explore breathwork. Approach it with an open heart and a sprinkle of curiosity. It can be a fantastic support as you navigate the twists and turns of perimenopause.

Bottom line? Breathwork is like a best friend during perimenopause—always there to help you find balance, feel amazing and embrace the changes happening in your body and mind. So, why not give it a shot and let your breath guide you on a journey of self-discovery and empowerment during perimenopause and beyond?

If you are interested in a FREE 1:1 20 breathwork session contact Polly Warren at info@pollywarren.com.

Notes:

CHAPTER THIRTY FIVE
Reduce the Pressure: Understanding and Looking After Your Blood Pressure During Perimenopause
By Susannah Alexander

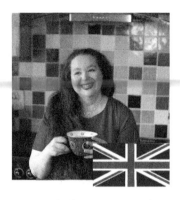

Bio: I'm Susannah, a size-friendly nutritional therapist with a first-class honours degree. I am an experienced educator and speaker who is passionate about helping people understand and make friends with their bodies at every size and removing weight stigma in healthcare. To learn more about me, my online blood pressure course and my wellness breaks in the Scottish Highlands please visit me at www.nodramanutrition.co.uk.

Business: No Drama Nutrition
Website: www.nodramanutrition.co.uk

Before perimenopause high blood pressure is a relatively rare problem for women. However, during and after perimenopause things can change. Perhaps you thought this was an issue that only affected older men with beer guts. Perhaps you are asking yourself why this is happening or perhaps you are not sure what you can do other than (or as well as) taking several medications for life. If any of this is familiar, this chapter is for you.

High blood pressure is often described as a 'silent killer' because most people will have no symptoms. Around 30-50% of women will develop it before the age of 60. Having high blood pressure after menopause may increase your risk of a heart attack by up to five times as well as putting you at increased risk of dementia and of death from any cause. But in this case knowledge really is power because high blood pressure is the biggest modifiable risk factor for heart disease.

Not everyone can modify their blood pressure. Some people inherit high blood pressure and there is no known way to change that other than taking medication. However, there's good news too. For those who can influence their blood pressure even small changes can make a huge difference. Lowering diastolic pressure by 5 points reduces the chances of heart attack by 20% and stroke by 32%. If you're in your 40s or early 50s now is a really good time to be reading this because the earlier you can take action, the lower your risk of disease is likely to be.

In this chapter I'm going to explain what those words and numbers mean, how to avoid misdiagnosis and what you can do to look after your blood pressure if you are diagnosed with hypertension.

What is blood pressure?

Blood pressure is a measure of the force your body uses to

pump blood around the body. The higher the pressure the more force is being used. Blood pressure numbers are shown as one figure over another, for example 120/70 mmHg. The mmHg stands for 'milligrams of mercury' which is the unit of measurement for blood pressure.

The larger number on top is called systolic pressure and is the amount of pressure exerted when the muscles in your heart contract. The smaller number on the bottom is called diastolic pressure and refers to the amount of pressure when your heart muscles relax. The top number is thought to be the best predictor of long-term disease and the one to watch.

Knowing your Numbers

High blood pressure, also known as hypertension, is currently defined as being greater than 140/90 mmHg. Either one or both the numbers may exceed this level.

In the UK the blood pressure thresholds are as follows. *(See table on next page)*

90/60mmHg or lower	Low blood pressure. Not usually considered a problem but worth checking if you often feel dizzy.
90/60-120/80mmHg	Ideal blood pressure.
120/80-140/90mmHg	Prehypertension. You don't have high blood pressure but you could be heading in that direction. This is a good time to consider taking action.
140/90mmHg or higher	Hypertension. You have high blood pressure and should consider lifestyle changes and/or medication.

Why is this a Peri issue?

Blood pressure issues affect women more as they reach perimenopause and menopause. This is likely to be influenced by a number of factors, many of which are beyond your control. These include:

- Changes in nervous system activity which can promote inflammation and oxidative stress. These in turn can damage blood vessel walls.
- Arteries can become thicker and stiffer. When blood flows through them with force they are less flexible resulting in greater pressure.
- One of oestrogen's effects is to dilute blood vessels. Falling levels of oestrogen means this does not happen as much, forcing blood to flow through a narrower space and increasing the pressure. However, HRT has not been demonstrated consistently to lower blood pressure. It is thought that testosterone may be involved as well.
- Some women become more sensitive to salt after menopause. This means that there is excess salt in the bloodstream, which can lead to fluid retention, which in turn raises blood pressure.

So, if you do develop hypertension, it's important not to feel guilty or think that you caused the problem. That's rubbish! However, that doesn't mean there's nothing you can do.

There is plenty of positive action you can take.

How to get diagnosed correctly

Hypertension should never be diagnosed from one reading. Your blood pressure can vary quite a bit depending on a number of factors. Imagine that you have run to the doctor in a state of stress after eating a cheese sandwich and a packet of crisps! Of course, your blood pressure will be higher than someone who is totally relaxed at their appointment, is well rested and has not eaten for a few hours.

In order to get the right results for you either at home or with a health practitioner you should:

- Make sure the correct sized cuff is used. If you have big arms like me, a standard cuff will give you a false high reading. Insist on the right size or you may get misdiagnosed.
- Don't do cardiovascular exercise right before you measure.
- Try to be relaxed when your blood pressure is measured. Think of something lovely and remember to breathe.
- Don't eat salty food or drink lots of water before measuring your pressure.

If you have a high blood pressure reading at the doctor's don't panic! You should be given a blood pressure monitor to use at home. When you are more relaxed in your own environment you are more likely to get a reading that truly represents your situation.

But if blood pressure is still a concern here are some actions you can take to support this crucial aspect of your health.

PLEASE NOTE: this section contains dietary recommendations that are safe and effective for the general population, but some may not be right for you. Speak with a health professional about your specific needs if you're planning to change how you eat or supplement your food, particularly if you are using medication.

DASH your way to lower blood pressure

In 2018 the US News and Health Report ranked a DASH-type diet as the best overall diet (out of 38 diets) and the best for heart health. In comparison to the general population following a DASH-type diet involves consuming:

- More fruits and vegetables
- More whole grains
- Fewer non-beneficial fats
- A similar amount of meat and dairy
- Fewer refined sugars
- Less alcohol

Further modifications to the original DASH diet which have been shown to help are:

- Reducing salt (this happens naturally when you eat fewer manufactured foods)
- Eating full-fat rather than reduced fat dairy
- Not drinking fruit juice

Following a DASH-type approach can show benefit in as little as 2 weeks. The higher your blood pressure was to start with the more it has been shown to help.

Key Minerals: Sodium, Potassium and Magnesium

We need some sodium in our diets, but the average Brit is eating too much. Most of the excess comes from manufactured foods so reducing these is an excellent step.

Incidentally, sodium and salt are not the same thing. Food labels may only list the sodium content of the food in order to convince you that their product is low in salt. To discover the true salt content of a food, multiply the sodium by 2.5. The adult upper limit for dietary salt is 6g so you are aiming for less than or equal to this level.

However, salt and sodium aren't the whole story. Sodium's partner in the body is potassium. Together they affect fluid balance, kidney function and the nervous system.

Sodium reduction is more effective when combined with increasing dietary potassium. This happens naturally when you eat more fruit and vegetables. In particular, be sure to include:

- Avocados
- Tomatoes
- Orange fruit such as peaches apricots and melons
- Bananas

- Potatoes

The third mineral that may play a vital role in blood pressure is magnesium. Magnesium is thought to help blood vessels to relax, creating a greater area for blood flow. It may also play a role in keeping blood vessels healthy by reducing inflammation and acting as an antioxidant.

Having enough magnesium in your diet has been shown to be helpful for blood pressure in the long term and becomes more helpful the longer you maintain sufficient levels. The recommended daily amount for women is 320 mg a day but it's generally safe and may be beneficial to have up to 500mg. If you decide to supplement and you are also experiencing insomnia you may find magnesium glycinate helpful.

The best dietary sources of magnesium are almonds, cashew nuts, Brazil nuts and English walnuts. You can also enjoy:

- Brown rice
- Figs
- Dates
- Sweetcorn
- Edamame
- Spinach
- Plain yoghurt
- Kidney beans
- Avocados
- Bananas
- Salmon

3 is the Magic Number

You have probably heard about 'good fats'. 'Good' in the context of blood pressure means fat sources high in omega-3. This essential fat may help to make blood vessels more elastic and help to prevent artery-blocking plaques forming. For some people getting plenty of omega-3 (between 2 and 4g a day) may be more clinically significant than reducing alcohol, exercising or even salt reduction.

The foods with the highest and best converting omega-3 levels are oily fish. You can eat up to 2 portions a week and up to 4 if you are no longer trying to conceive. Consider including smaller freshwater fish such as sardines, mackerel and trout as these are less exposed to mercury than salmon and tuna. If you don't eat fish, you may need to consider a supplement. Or add 2 teaspoons of flaxseed a day to your diet. Be sure to choose a reputable supplement brand and always ensure your fish oil comes with Vitamin E, as fish oils can degrade easily.

Food is of course only one piece of the dietary picture. Remember to stay well hydrated. Enjoy as much water and herbal tea as you can. For blood pressure, tea and coffee are probably fine.

Alcohol is another story. Many studies suggest that having more than 1 drink a day can be a risk factor for high blood pressure, particularly if you binge drink or drink away from meals. If you like a drink, your best option is to enjoy one glass of red wine with a meal, as this may have a small benefit for heart health.

Which Exercise is Best?

Being physically active has a huge range of health benefits and may help with blood pressure too. But which exercise is most effective?

HIIT training has been shown to benefit systolic blood pressure in a shorter space of time than steady-state cardiovascular exercise, but it may not be right for everyone. If you already have high blood pressure it could even be quite harmful as it can push up your blood pressure rapidly in the short term. You probably need professional support in order to work at the right intensity for you and avoid injury. If you are newer to exercise you may not even be able to reach the necessary intensity.

Luckily many studies show that instead of cardiovascular exercise, which often shows negligible benefit, activities such as Tai Chi yoga and Nia show consistent benefit, possibly because these exercises have a meditative component and therefore help with stress management. Managing stress is extremely important for regulating blood pressure. While you can't eliminate stress in your life it's important to identify what really pushes your buttons and come up with some strategies to manage your response.

A word about medication

Even if you do everything possible to live a blood-pressure friendly life you may still need medication. This is nothing to be ashamed of and you haven't failed. If you need to do this to take care of yourself, do it!

If you want to understand more about your medication nutrition, or any other aspect of your blood pressure health, please get in touch.

Finally relax and breathe. You've got this.

There is so much more to say about each of the subjects in this chapter as well as hints, tips and recipes to share. I have packed them into a user-friendly 21-day online course. If you or anyone you know could benefit from this, just scan the QR code. I know it works, because I've done it myself and achieved great results.

Journal prompts:

What thoughts, ideas and feelings does the term 'high blood pressure' bring up for you? Has reading this chapter changed any of your preconceptions? If so, how?

What are three things you already do to look after your blood pressure?

What are three things you could improve or add in order to support your blood pressure even more?

What might be the barriers to making these upgrades?

What could you do to overcome these?

What additional knowledge, resources or help do you need to support blood pressure health, and where can you find it?

What one action can you take right now that would make a meaningful difference?

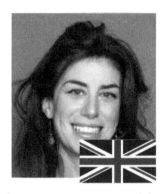

CHAPTER THIRTY SIX
Navigating Your Relationship with Food and Body Image During the Perimenopause by Marcelle Rose

Bio: Marcelle is a BANT Registered Nutritionist, Health Coach and Master Practitioner of Eating Disorders. Her expertise lies in helping women overcome emotional eating, binge eating, bulimia and restrictive eating behaviours so they can make peace with their body, heal their relationship with food and reclaim their life. Marcelle consults with clients nationwide and worldwide bringing together nutritional therapy, the psychology of eating and behaviour change coaching. Keen to support women however she can with food and body challenges, Marcelle runs a free Facebook group community, The food Freedom Collective.

Business: Marcelle Rose - Emotional & Disordered Eating Specialist
Website: www.marcellerosenutrition.co.uk

For countless women, the menopause transition is a pivotal time when challenges around food and body image resurface or worsen. For others, this life stage marks the initial onset of these difficulties.

344

So, what prompts these shifts, and how can we as women make peace with food and our body and protect ourselves from the potential risks?

Just as you may have explored in the earlier sections of this book, the journey through midlife brings about significant shifts in our body. Most notable are the ebb and flow of rollercoasting oestrogen, eventually giving way to a notable decline alongside dropping progesterone levels. These alterations in our hormonal landscape lead to a multitude of changes in our biology, affecting our physical, psychological, and emotional well-being. As a result, this life phase can have a profound influence on our relationship with food and body image where the dynamics of our eating habits and how we view ourselves may change significantly.

As you approach this life stage, you might have already observed changes in your own eating behaviours such as persistent dieting, restriction of food groups or calorie counting. You may label yourself an emotional eater, or perhaps you binge eat or feel out of control around food.

For countless women, the menopause transition is a pivotal time when challenges around food and body image resurface or worsen. For others, this life stage marks the initial onset of these difficulties. **So, what prompts these shifts, and how can we as women make peace with food and our body and protect ourselves from the potential risks during this time?**

A Means of Coping

Disordered eating behaviours can often develop as a coping mechanism when life feels overwhelming and out of control. The symptoms that often accompany menopause – such as anxiety, depression, sleep disturbances, and a sense of cognitive decline – can create the perfect storm. Simultaneously, many of us find ourselves juggling the responsibilities of caring for elderly parents and adjusting to our grown children leaving home. For some women this phase coincides with the breakdown of their marriage adding to sensations of loss, change, and overwhelm.

Evolution of Weight & Body Appearance

Change in body shape and weight is common as we navigate the perimenopause. New oestrogen lows in addition to declining progesterone can cause a metabolic change that leads to weight gain around the middle. During this time, we will experience a fifteen percent drop in our metabolic rate (This is your calories burned while at rest) partly due to the reduced ability to hold on to muscle but is also due to the shift to insulin resistance. This is a major player in abdominal weight gain and women who have previously had PCOS (polycystic ovarian syndrome) are even more at risk developing menopausal insulin resistance and weight gain. It's also worth noting that while thyroid disease develops independently of the perimenopause, the perimenopausal phase can exacerbate the autoimmune condition Hashimoto's due to a recalibration of the immune system at this time.

Many women find it distressing to discover that what they were doing before -in terms of diet and exercise -is no longer working for them. This is when dietary restraint may emerge whether it be trying calorie deficit diets, fasting or eliminating food groups such as carbs or fats.

Sleep Quality & Quantity

Lack of sleep, which often goes hand in hand with perimenopause due to night sweats or anxiety, also influences our eating patterns. When sleep quality diminishes, it affects both our appetite and the choices we make about what to eat. The hormones that control our sense of fullness, leptin, decrease, while the hunger-inducing hormone, ghrelin, increases. This combination means that we are more likely to crave less nutritious foods.

Furthermore, inadequate sleep has multiple repercussions. It affects mood and weakens our ability to handle stress. With diminished energy and motivation, the task of preparing a balanced meal can become overwhelming. This often results in a greater inclination to turn to food for a quick energy boost and perhaps comfort.

The Cortisol Connection

Change in body shape can be attributed, in part, to the intricate interplay between physiology and levels of the stress hormone, cortisol. These shifts can also influence changes in body composition, altering where the body tends to store fat.

Cortisol, one of your key stress hormones, comes into play when you need to respond to immediate danger. Its effects on your body involve boosting your heart rate, raising blood pressure, and making more glucose available in your bloodstream. All of this is geared to provide energy for your muscles for a 'fight or flight' scenario.

However, problems arise if you are in a regular state of stress and continually activating cortisol. This can cause a cascade of issues including fatigue, feelings of anxiousness, and sugar cravings. Crucially, chronic stress reduces how responsive your body is to insulin and impacts its ability to effectively process the glucose present in your blood.

Insulin's Role

In addition to insulin's role in controlling your blood glucose levels, it also plays a part in managing your appetite. When you eat, your brain notices the rise in insulin levels in your body, leading to a reduction in hunger. Certain studies suggest that if we develop insulin resistance, meaning that insulin's effectiveness is diminished, it might struggle to reach the brain and perform its job of reducing hunger.

Brain Chemicals & Cravings

During a regular menstrual cycle, the decrease in oestrogen levels that occurs before menstruation also brings about a reduction in the brain chemicals dopamine and serotonin. This physiological change often results in intense sugar cravings and a heightened appetite just prior to the onset of your period. In the context of perimenopause, the erratic fluctuations of oestrogen can similarly trigger powerful cravings linked to the diminished levels of these crucial brain chemicals.

Serotonin, often referred to as the 'happy hormone,' acts as a potent mood-enhancing neurotransmitter. Meanwhile, dopamine, is responsible for generating feelings of reward and pleasure, each plays a pivotal role. A decline in both dopamine and serotonin levels makes us more inclined to seek out foods that provide a dopamine surge and feelings of comfort and pleasure, for some this leads to emotional eating and bingeing behaviour.

Why Dieting Doesn't Help

Perimenopausal women often turn to dieting because they're dissatisfied with their body, however this rarely improves their body image. Furthermore, a history of dieting can exacerbate concerns about body and weight during midlife. Although not directly tied to menopause, multiple dieting attempts affect our set point which acts like a thermostat for the weight range that our body is happiest at. This set point tends to increase each time a diet is attempted as your body strives to regulate itself.

Dietary restraint is a significant trigger for the most prevalent of the eating disorders, Binge Eating Disorder (BED). It affects one in fifty people officially -but the figures are likely to be higher in reality. Many people may suffer with the challenges of binge eating without necessarily meeting the criteria for BED yet will still experience a great deal distress and a constant sense of shame and guilt.

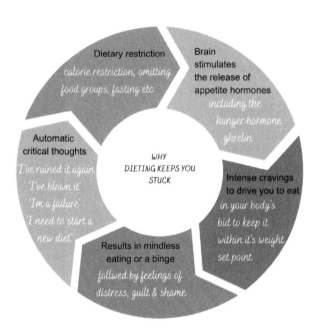

So, What Can You Do About It?

Whether you find your thoughts entirely consumed by food, your body and weight, leaving no mental space for anything else, or you engage in food restriction, compensatory behaviours, emotionally eat or binge to the point of distress, it's important to know that it is possible to create change in your life.

Where To Start?

I recommend beginning with the following simple steps. Your life might already feel pretty overwhelming, so it's important not to add in more complications right now. However, do not underestimate the potential of these steps— they can make a real impact, and you are likely to experience benefits early on. For additional resources and detailed guidance on these, download my complimentary guide 'Breaking the Cycle.'

Now, let's get into the initial three steps:

1. Regulate – establish regular eating patterns

One of the first things I address when working with my clients is their eating patterns. Contrary to common beliefs about eating, consuming three balanced meals and incorporating snacks if and when needed, can significantly impact your body's biology and help to address the physiological reasons for cravings. Starting to establish a consistent eating routine, will help your body to become accustomed to receiving energy at specific times, leading to a reduction in hunger and cravings. Consequently, you're less likely to seek out foods that provide quick but short-lived energy and become more capable of making mindful decisions around food. If this feels far away from where you are now, start by adding in one new meal at a time. For example, if your eating is currently chaotic and you are skipping proper meals – first just begin by introducing a small breakfast and build on that over time.

2. Evaluate - develop a better understanding of your body's appetite cues

You were born knowing how to eat what your body needed. Over time, you have learnt how to manually override these instincts. Using the hunger scale (below) regularly, will help you to feel more in touch with your hunger, fullness and satiety signals. At the beginning and after you have eaten, notice any physical signs; For example, if your stomach is rumbling or your mouth is watering - do bear in mind the signs may be more subtle than this. Don't decide anything about yourself and your hunger. Just notice where you are. Slowing down your eating can really help with this as you will allow time for your brain to catch up with your stomach.

It is still important to stick to your regular eating patterns even if you don't feel hungry at certain times – it takes time to tune in effectively especially if you have been dieting and overriding your appetite cues for years.

The Hunger Scale

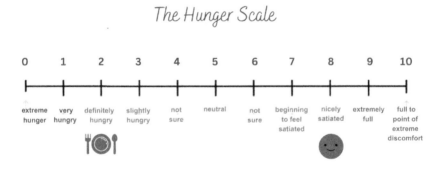

3. Satisfy – incorporate snacks with intention

Snacks will alleviate true hunger, but how do you know if you're experiencing a craving and not true hunger? A tell-tale sign of a craving is that you feel a nearly uncontrollable need to eat a specific food. On the other hand, you can choose to consume a specific food at a set point in time. Cravings tend to be for specific foods and they can rage when your blood glucose levels are destabilised or if you have a particular emotional attachment to a food.

By listening to your body's signals, you can begin to pay attention to your hunger and energy levels throughout the day. On a practical note, be prepared with snacks in advance to have them readily available when needed. It's also essential to avoid waiting until you become over hungry before eating as this is far more likely to end in mindlessly eating something less helpful.

When it comes to the snacks themselves, choose nutrient-dense options to provide sustained energy and help keep your blood glucose stable. Where possible try a combination of protein, natural fats, and complex carbohydrates for example full fat natural yoghurt with berries, nuts and seeds and humous with oatcakes or veggie sticks.

Develop the Art of Self-Compassion

The idea of self-compassion is often misunderstood and commonly regarded as self-indulgent or a sign of weakness.

However, learning self-compassion has the science to back it up. It can make a profound difference to your overall wellbeing and self-esteem -positively impacting your eating behaviour and body image struggles, whilst supporting you through the challenges of perimenopause.

One of the key areas is self-kindness which is essentially being understanding with yourself and reducing self-criticism and blame. It allows you to see your own flaws with understanding and accept your imperfections. A helpful way to reframe negative critical thoughts about yourself is to think about what you would say to a good friend. Would you talk to them in the same way as yourself? What would you say to them in the same situation?

Let's take the example of the binge eating cycle –

You eat something you wish you hadn't or experienced a binge – your automatic thought is 'I've ruined it again' or 'I've blown it'.

A more compassionate response might be something like:
- *I notice that I have found this difficult, but I'm OK.*
- *I wonder what might have been going on for me to lead to this eating event?*
- *What might I be needing, to do something differently next time?*

Embracing self-compassion will play an integral role as you embark on your journey to heal your relationship with food and your body. The process isn't focused on achieving a 'flawless' diet or conforming to society's ideals of the 'perfect' body. Instead, it involves making small, incremental changes one day at a time whilst treating yourself with care, respect and kindness.

Scan the QR code to begin your journey to a healthier relationship with food today, using my free 4 step guide

Whether you're a lifelong dieter, a binge eater, or someone who struggles with food-related guilt and shame, I've created something that can help you. I've drawn on a decade's experience of working with women who struggle with emotional and disordered eating, to provide you with four actionable steps that you can begin to implement today.

'Breaking the cycle – your first steps to healing your relationship with food' is an essential resource for anyone who suffers from emotional or disordered eating

Journal prompts:

I am inspired to…

You are worthy of love, happiness and respect no matter your body size, weight or shape

CHAPTER THIRTY SEVEN
Radiant Skin Through Perimenopause:
Navigating Emotions for Holistic Beauty
By Sahar Hooti

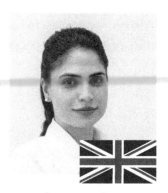

Bio: Meet Sahar, your holistic wellness guide specialising in perimenopause care, blending her roles as an Acupuncture Practitioner, Aromatherapist, and Advanced Skin Therapist. Sahar is a Heart Health advocate, recognising that true wellness starts from within. With a focus on mental well-being, she weaves a tapestry of health where vibrant skin is a reflection of flourishing circulation and overall vitality. Sahar offers both online consultations globally and in-person sessions at her clinic in the UK, empowered by her AromaAcu Therapy™ method and affiliation with the British Acupuncture Council.

Business: AcuCare Clinic
Website: https://acucareclinic.co.uk

"Beauty is everywhere, but sometimes we need a stroll in the garden to see it." - Rumi

Alright, picture this: Rumi, the Persian poet, was like the ultimate life coach, reminding us to find the good stuff right under our noses. We're diving into the world of 'perimenopause and skin', a topic I'm sure you all have questions about!

I'm Sahar, your guide on this journey. I've got Traditional Chinese Medicine (TCM)/Acupuncture in my pocket, a sprinkle of aromatherapy magic, the scoop on modern science, and beauty therapy skin care insights.

Before we start, I've got something juicy from my Persian roots. My mother, Parvin Keshavarz, a total queen, handled perimenopause like a boss. She told me, "Each stage of our life brings secret goodies, even if they're hiding." Imagine that, hidden blessings in all the chaos!

Ageing is a wild adventure, a treasure trove of lessons. Just like Mum said, perimenopause is like a mirror reflecting your journey- even the chapters you didn't plan.

Your skin's like a storybook, every line a tale of your laugh-out-loud moments, conquering dragons, and dancing in the rain. So here we are, with Mum's wisdom lighting our path. In this chapter, we're turning perimenopause into a masterpiece- where feelings and skin blend in perfect harmony.

Ready? Let's get into the nitty-gritty of how these two rebels come together during this crazy phase.

The Skin's Story: A Reflection of Emotions and Life's Chapters

Imagine your skin as a super cool journal, the kind that tells your story without you even speaking. Now, hold tight as we dive into the perimenopause whirlwind. Your skin's joining this adventure, flipping pages like crazy. It's your life story unfolding right there on your face. Every line's a chapter, each wrinkle a story. It's not just skin- no no no, it's your own personal best-seller!

Getting older is not just about counting candles on your cake; it's about owning each chapter. Every line on your face is a badge of honour, a medal for facing whatever life has thrown at you. It's like battle scars, but with a twist of elegance. Those lines, they're markers of wisdom earned. Your face? It's a walking storybook, telling tales of courage, love, heartbreaks and everything in between.

Unmasking the Connection Between Emotional Well-Being and Skin Health

Emotions
Emotions are not just a side dish in your life's buffet; they're the VIPs who sneak into your skin's party too. Take Stress for example. It's not just in your head; it's got a backstage pass to mess with your skin's glow. Think of it as your skin's personal drama queen.

And there's more. Traditional Chinese Medicine jumps in

with its two cents. We say emotions tango with vital energy (we call it Qi pronounced as Chee) and blood circulation. Our emotions initiate a secret convo between our heart and our skin. And here we are, caught in the middle of science and ancient wisdom, making sense of perimenopause and skin health!

Our Skin's Universal Essence

The Vital Role of the Skin: A Window into Inner Health and Holistic Well-Being

Skin, the lovely canvas of our bodies. It's a wonderful mirror that reflects what's inside. Your skin doesn't only show off your most recent sun-kissed tan or how well you wore that sparkly eyeshadow last night. No, it's a lot smarter than that. Your skin is the ultimate gossip queen; it reveals your underlying health secrets. If your body is holding an internal party, your skin is definitely invited.

Our skin is more than just the outside shell; it's a window into our whole health. Remember that time you ate too many greasy fries and woke up with a spot?

That's your skin giving you the side eye because of your food choices. Skin may disclose hormonal imbalances, dietary inadequacies, and even your stress levels. It's not just about spots and acne.

Let us now take a brief diversion to Traditional Chinese Medicine (TCM). For thousands of years, experts have been decoding the skin-health relationship. We believe that our skin is a literal reflection of our body's interior harmony. If your Qi (your body's energy flow) is flowing in a balanced manner, your skin will glow like a million little stars. However, if there is a Qi traffic bottleneck, expect breakouts, dry areas, and possibly even an unwanted wrinkle or two.

The Skin as a Mirror of the Body in TCM

Let us go deeper down the TCM rabbit hole. We take the phrase "you are what you eat" to an entirely new level. Every organ in your body, according to TCM, is linked to a specific portion of your face. It's like a hidden treasure map, with all the clues hidden in your skin. For example, Dark circles could be SOS signals from your kidneys. Is your liver acting up? Say welcome to breakouts on your brow and a portion of your forehead area.

Skin health is more than just vanity in the practice of TCM- it's a road map to your body's state of balance. We believe that when your internal systems are perfectly synced, your skin will sing "I'm Walking on Sunshine" (not literally, but you get the drift).

So remember, my fellow travellers in the land of radiant skin and well-being: your skin is more than just a gorgeous face- it's the ultimate truth-teller. If you treat it well, it will reveal your inner health goals.

Lungs: The Breath of Life and Skin's Silent Guardian

Understanding Traditional Chinese Medicine's Lung-Skin Connection

Let's take a deep breath of information, shall we? Your lungs are the unsung heroes of skin health in the world of Traditional Chinese Medicine (TCM). They are not only responsible for keeping you breathing; they are also the commanders of your skin's defence squad. How? Let us break it down.

According to TCM, our lungs are in charge of circulating Qi throughout our body. Consider it a cosmic FedEx delivery service that ensures life force reaches every nook and cranny. Guess where Qi likes to hang out. You've got it- your skin!

You can hear your skin say, "Hey, I'm loving this energy boost!" when your lungs are happy and performing their Qi delivery dance. That's when your skin looks radiant and vibrant. However, if your lungs have a meltdown, it disrupts the energy flow and causes your skin to act like a grumpy adolescent. Acne, dullness, and even premature ageing are possible outcomes.

The Lungs' Role in Managing Perimenopausal Changes: Breathing Through Transitions

Let us now address the elephant in the room: Perimenopause. It's a rollercoaster of emotions, and your lungs are on high alert. Why? Because your body is going through a significant hormonal transition around this time, and guess who's tryingto keep things balanced? Yep, those superhuman lungs of yours.

Perimenopause can feel like the wildest party you've ever been to, with your lungs playing DJ and trying to keep the beat steady. But here's the catch: they require extra love and attention throughout this period.

You see, stress loves to gatecrash the party, and it messes with your lung's energy flow. Suddenly, your skin might be shouting, "Why, oh why, are you doing this to me?" Breakouts, sensitivity, and dryness might make an appearance.

So, what's the secret recipe? Well, for starters, deep breathing is like a lung spa day. It helps release stress, keep the Qi flowing, and tell your skin, "Hey, we're in this together."

Emotional Beauty Therapy: The Healing Power of Emotions on Skin

Let's talk about emotions now. Those little powerhouses that can make you want to dance one minute and pull your hair out the next. The twist is that emotions are backstage magicians, and your skin is the stage. This dance takes front stage during perimenopause, and boy, does it have an effect on your complexion!

Stress, anxiety, and even those "Where did I put my keys?"

moments may all send signals to your skin faster than a text message. How? It's almost as though they had their own hotline. Cortisol, our stress hormone, is released by the body when you are stressed. And, guess what? Cortisol and your skin don't exactly greet each other warmly. It's the equivalent of inviting your least favourite relative to a family gathering.

As a result, stress can cause your skin to become irritated. Breakouts, flare-ups, redness, and skin sagginess etc may decide to join in on the fun. But here's the thing: you don't have to be a stoic superhero to succeed. Emotions are a natural aspect of the human experience, and they are not going away. What counts is how you move through this dance.

Connecting Emotions with Skin Manifestations: Insights from Traditional Chinese Medicine

Now, let's shift gears and tap into TCM's ancient knowledge. Emotions and skin are like old friends who catch up over tea. According to TCM, each emotion has its own energy that flows through certain pathways (*meridians* located over major neural pathways) in your body. So, when emotions are enjoying their own mini funfair, they can also alter the radiance of your skin.

Remember that stress we talked about earlier? In TCM, it's like a roadblock for your Qi. And when Qi can't move freely, your skin might decide to put up a protest. Your skin is saying, "Hey, I need some breathing room too!"

This is when TCM comes to the rescue and offers its own toolkit of solutions. It offers a spa day for your Qi, with everything from acupuncture to herbs. I actually help my patients with the magic of aromatherapy instead of herbs, but you can also achieve great results with just acupuncture. When your energy is in sync, your skin says, "Cheers to that!"

A Holistic Approach to Ageless Beauty: Bringing Ancient Wisdom and Modern Science Together

Beauty Inside Out: How Nutritious Foods and Hydration Nourish and Illuminate the Skin

Let's share some skin-care tips that don't involve magical potions or magic wands. Consider your skin to be a garden, and what you feed it has a direct impact on how it grows. During perimenopause, your skin deserves an extra dose of TLC. How? Through your plate!

Nutrient-rich foods aren't just good for your waistline; they're skin's besties too.

What are omega-3 fatty acids?

They're like the rockstars of skin health, fighting inflammation and locking in moisture. And antioxidants? They're the bodyguards against those sneaky free radicals. So, load up on berries, leafy greens, and those yummy avocados.

But don't forget about the glass half full- literally. Hydration is the happy pill for your skin. It gives your skin a shot of energy. Water washes out toxins, plumps up your skin cells, and maintains your bright glow. Carry that water bottle about like it's your secret weapon!

Natural and Timeless Combination: The Synergy of Aromatherapy and Acupuncture- or as I call it 'AromaAcu Therapy™'

Hold onto your hats, because we're diving into a world of scents and sensations. Say hello to aromatherapy, the ultimate soul-soothing spa treatment that you can have anywhere and anytime. Consider it a one-way ticket to serenity.

Aromatherapy is more than just pleasant aromas; it also promotes emotional well-being. Essential oils like lavender and chamomile are like a lullaby for your senses, calming your mind and in turn, reflecting on your skin. A gentle reminder that tranquillity and radiance are BFFs.

With the help of my professional Aromatherapy background, I started using tailored magical healing blends combined with traditional Acupuncture for my patients. The effectiveness of the results were so evident through this treatment combo. Patients were floating out of my clinic room!

Aromatic plants have been hailed as skin's sidekicks for centuries. From promoting circulation to harmonising energy flow, aromatherapy and TCM are the dynamic duo your skin never knew it needed. Just make sure you learn how to use them properly as they can also be harmful to your health. The safest way to reset is to just apply a drop of essential oil onto a tissue and just inhale. Might as well practise a good breathing method at the same time. I recommend 'Box Breathing'. Google it and find what works best for you!

The Harmony of Cosmetic Acupuncture: Merging Aesthetics and Healing

Unveiling Natural Radiance: The Face Lifting Magic of Cosmetic Acupuncture

Let's delve into the fascinating field of cosmetic acupuncture-where beauty meets ancient wisdom. Consider this: microscopic, hair-thin needles performing a rejuvenation symphony on your skin. It's not just about looking for the illusive fountain of youth; it's also about boosting your skin's natural vitality.

Cosmetic acupuncture isn't about changing who you are; it's about recognising and appreciating the work of art that is you! What about those acupuncture needles? I hear you! Well, you don't feel them if that's what you mean, they're there to increase blood flow and Qi and restore your skin's radiance. Let us now add a dash of science to this ancient art form. Cosmetic acupuncture has been demonstrated in studies to increase collagen production, minimise the appearance of fine wrinkles, and even improve skin suppleness.

It's a boost of confidence with every needle tap!

A Bridge Between Traditions: Merging Beauty Therapy and Chinese Medicine

Meet the ultimate power couple: Beauty Therapy and Traditional Chinese Medicine.

It's like a love story where each partner brings out the best in the other. Through my personal and professional experience, Beauty Therapy, with its modern expertise, teams up so well with the ancient wisdom of TCM, and together, they're rewriting the rules of skin care.

Consider it an art form in which ancient practices such as the popular Gua Sha (pronounced as Gwah Sha) Facial and current technologies coexist for the ultimate well-being of your skin. My Beauty Therapy combo treatments don't just focus on the surface; it's about diving deep and nurturing your skin from within. And guess what? TCM is the guiding compass, ensuring that every touch, every technique, aligns with your body's natural rhythm.This powerful combination serves as a reminder that beauty is more than just skin deep; it is a reflection of your overall well-being. The tradition of Chinese Medicine merges effortlessly with the innovation of Beauty Therapy to create a symphony that celebrates you in all your brilliant splendour.

A Glowing Routine for Perimenopause Skin Care:

The Unfolding Journey: How Perimenopause and Menopause Affect the Skin

Welcome to the heart of skin care- where self-care becomes

an art and your skin blossoms with timeless radiance. Perimenopause and menopause bring a shift in the skin's landscape, a transformation that's written in the language of your body. Hormones dance their wild tango, and your skin? Well, it's the canvas where this dance unfolds.

Dryness? You might find your skin feeling a tad parched. Wrinkles? They're little badges of wisdom, showcasing your life's journey. But don't panic; there's no need to go all combat mode. It's about embracing this new chapter, understanding what your skin needs, and giving it a dose of nourishment that's second to none.

So, let's talk about rituals- those small everyday rituals that make you feel like the queen you are. Your skin, too, deserves to be treated like royalty. It's time to reveal a brilliant regimen that combines the wisdom of tradition with the modern wonder of science.

First and foremost, cleanse. It's like a new beginning, washing away the day's events and allowing your skin to breathe. But here's the thing: being kind is the goal. No need to go all gladiator on your skin; it's about kindness, the kind that says, "Hey, I've got your back, or should I say, your face!" Never ever skip this step before you go to sleep!

Then comes hydration. Consider your skin to be a desert in need of rain. Moisturisers, like rainfall, quench the thirst of your skin. What's more, we're talking about nutrient-rich moisturisers (preferably aromatherapy based) that your skin will savour like a fine wine.

Not to mention the superhero combination of sunscreen and antioxidants (such as Vitamin C). They act as bodyguards for your skin, shielding it from the sun's rays and those pesky free radicals. This daytime combination is essential for avoiding skin cancer, severe burns, fine lines and wrinkles, sun spots, and collagen depletion. When you combine sunscreen with vitamin C you effectively double the skin protection effects. Apply the Vitamin C before your moisturiser, and then apply sunscreen as your final step.

Beyond the Surface: Understanding Skin's Absorption and Impact on Our Well-Being

Here's a fun fact: your skin is like a sponge, soaking in everything you put on it. But, it's not just about beauty products; it's about the air you breathe, the water you splash, and the love you radiate. Your skin is the gatekeeper, deciding what gets in and what stays out.

Have you ever heard of "clean" beauty? It's similar to asking your skin to a luxury event when only the best ingredients are used. But this is where science comes in, ensuring that clean is also effective. One of my favourite ingredients that I use within my bespoke and handmade skin care prescriptions is *Hyaluronic Acid*. I believe this is where science and nature collaborate to provide you the best of both worlds.

Mindful Choices: The Science-Backed Importance of Clean and Natural Skin Care

It's time to put on our detective hats and understand ingredient lists. I'm talking paraben-free, sulphate-free, and all those "frees" that make you and your skin feel happy. But here's the catch: not everything labelled "natural" is actually skin-friendly. This is where education comes in. A discerning buyer looks behind the label and asks, "Hey, what's really inside this bottle?"

Out of my own frustration, my handmade and bespoke skin care range was born. It's free of any nasties and is only made with organic natural ingredients used by many women around the world. I feel very honoured and humbled that I have this opportunity to raise awareness about the importance of choosing smart and healthy skin care.

Gazing Toward Tomorrow: A Future Filled with Radiant Beauty and Self-Acceptance

Dear beautiful reader,

You've embarked on a remarkable journey- one of self-discovery, skin loving, and appreciating the differences that make you uniquely you. You have in your hands a guide that goes beyond skin deep, from the wisdom of ancient Chinese medicine to the wonder of aromatherapy and the insights of modern science.

Remember that you are not alone as you journey through

371

perimenopause and menopause.Your skin, this canvas of life's chapters, tells a story of resilience, growth, and wisdom. Let this chapter be your compass, guiding you through the beauty of emotions, the science of skin, and the harmony of holistic care. Let this be the push that you needed to remind you of the importance of *holistic self-care*, ie taking care of your mental health and keeping your skin happy as a result.

And as you go forth, remember the power of choice. Choose self-care, choose wisdom, and choose a journey that celebrates the ageless essence within you.

You are a work of art, a symphony of experiences, and a glowing soul. May your path be illuminated by the radiance of self-assurance, the warmth of self-acceptance, and the promise of a future that is uniquely and beautifully yours.

Last but not least, I'd like to raise awareness about something very important. Note that not every Acupuncture Practitioner is a Beauty Therapist or an Aromatherapist. The unique approach presented in this chapter is the result of my diverse educational background and training. When seeking the services of Acupuncturists, Beauty Therapists, or Aromatherapists, ensure they hold proper qualifications (look for a degree in Traditional Chinese Medicine / Acupuncture) and memberships with reputable organisations such as The British Acupuncture council.

Look out for # AcuWarrior # TheHootiMethod
Feel free to tag me #AcuCareClinicInternational

Online consultations and 1-2-1 Health & Skin Care
Workshops are available worldwide.

I currently offer clinic visits at my UK practice in the lovely
Hampshire areas: Southsea and Waterlooville.

Wishing you health, joy, success, beautiful skin, and harmony,

Sahar xo

For personalised guidance and consultations,
reach out through the QR code

Chapter Notes and Reflections:

As you journey through the insights and wisdom of this chapter, take a moment to reflect on how each section resonates with your own experiences and aspirations. Use this space to jot down thoughts, questions, or even your own "aha!" moments that arise as you explore the connection between emotions, skin health, and holistic well-being. Feel free to write down any questions you'd like to ask me during a potential consultation, so we can dive deeper into your unique journey. Let your notes be a testament to your commitment to embracing your ageless essence and nurturing your radiant self.

"Each stage of our life brings secret goodies, even if they're hiding."-
Parvin Keshavarz

CHAPTER THIRTY EIGHT
The Power of Strength
Throughout Menopause
by Nikki Faldo

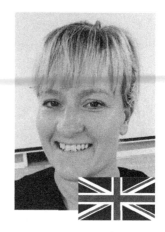

Bio: I'm Nikki, a Health and Wellness Coach specialising in Strength and Conditioning, nutrition, sleep and recovery, and Peri to Post Menopause health and wellbeing. I help women improve strength both physically and mentally, by taking an informed whole health approach that fits around your lifestyle to enable you to enjoy benefits such as weight loss, more energy, increased confidence and of course empowerment throughout menopause.

Business: EMPOWER - Strength Throughout Menopause
Website: https://instabook.io/landing/mindbodystrong
Facebook: https://www.facebook.com/nikki.hughes.357

So why strength?

I know firsthand how strength focused movement can make you stronger. Not just physically but mentally. A strong able, body will lead your mind that way too. I promise.

My chapter is a focus on strength training throughout menopause, not just perhaps the more obvious benefits it can bring, but all the ways we can be affected for the better.

So rather than just throw a ton of science facts your way however (that might come later), here's a little about me and my story to get us going. I experienced childhood trauma when I was 7. My father was mentally and physically abusive to my mother and it eventually got so bad that one night I tried to intervene and witnessed a violent situation.

As a teenager I turned to sport and exercise to help me through life as I was extremely unsociable in other settings, certainly wasn't willing to talk at that point and struggled immensely with self confidence, feelings of abandonment and let's just say my communication skills weren't great. Physical activity (of many forms) helped me immensely and at 17 I was offered a job as a Gym Instructor which I jumped at. My opportunity to help others as I had been helped by my coaches.

Throughout my career in gyms, I was never confident or comfortable in my body, always feeling larger than the other girls, fellow PTs and coaches. I experienced negative comments at various stages of my life. Even at my fittest at the end of my basic training in the British Army I was told I was "overweight" and may not pass out successfully (according to BMI...).

But I have always kept going, knowing and experiencing first hand all the other benefits that come not just from exercise, but from challenging my body, and therefore my mind and what it can try to tell me.

Fast forward to now and all of a sudden I have been in the health and fitness industry for over 27 years. I found myself realising more and more the benefits of strength training for all populations. However 6 years ago I started to specialise in training pre and post menopausal women.

As I have aged, so have my clients and I began hearing more and more about not just the obvious symptoms of menopause such as the flushes and brain fog, but the emotions, the life changes, job losses, relationship break ups and most of all, the total loss of self-confidence and self-love. Although I couldn't yet relate to symptoms, HRT options and preferences at that time, I could certainly relate to the self-love being lost and finding the strength to carry on at times seeming somewhat impossible.

Knowing what I knew (and do now even more) about how movement had helped me through some incredibly tough times mindset wise, I wanted to share my knowledge and experiences with these ladies and help bring back their self worth. I wanted to show them just what they are capable of, and of course be able to support them with as much knowledge as possible to provide the what's, whys and hows to back it all up!

So that's what I did, already a certified Nutrition Coach,

Personal Trainer, Strength and Conditioning Coach with MANY years of experience, I threw myself into further education around the menopause.

I am now in perimenopause myself and on HRT, and I not only resonate but can feel the benefits all the time of keeping a focus on continuing to build not just physical strength but resilience too.

But today I am here to focus on the strength side of things specifically. So, let's take a look at the physical stuff first, what happens to our muscles, bones and joints in menopause?

Around 30 years of age, our bodies will begin to change thanks to a process called sarcopenia. This is when our muscle mass will start deteriorating and we can lose up to 3-5% of our muscle mass each decade.... This rate will speed up after 65 years of age.

During menopause when we can experience a drop in oestrogen, this will also affect our muscle and bone mass negatively. The risk of osteoporosis (weakened bones, meaning more fragile) also increases. Strength/resistance focused movement can slow down the onset of both of these by promoting the maintenance and increase of lean muscle mass and bone density.

But how are you supposed to start to squeeze this into your life, what even is resistance training? You hate the thought of the gym, don't have an extra 5-6 hours in your week and wouldn't have a clue where to start.

Well the good news is that you can get started at home, even 20 mins of bodyweight focused movement twice a week is adequate to get you started and reaping the benefits.

Menopause can be a time where lots of women stop moving completely. Experiencing increased fatigue, lacking body confidence due to weight gain, pelvic health challenges, embarrassing sweats... the list goes on all making regular movement seem much less appetising so making it as easy as possible to get going is all important.

So what about our weight?

The amount of lean muscle mass we have will affect the health of our metabolism (think how well your body uses the energy/calories you put into it). If we look after your muscle mass your muscles will look after you. A healthy metabolism equals healthy, confident, less chance of injury, priceless independence as we age, the benefits go on and on!

But, it's not all about the muscles. Strength training will also improve cognitive health. By challenging and improving motor skills you can move more efficiently and confidently, and change your shape for the long term. I bet this isn't something your favourite diet influencer has told you!

Having worked with so many women throughout menopause specifically now, I see the other benefits that are not seen, or not at first anyway. Yes when my clients first chat with me there is a common feeling of lack of confidence and self-worth, in fact as sad as it is the statement " I don't like myself" or worse is unfortunately a common one to hear. Yes, these ladies want to lose a stubborn menopause belly initially, lose x amount of weight, be the weight they were when they were 30…

And of course I listen.

But as we get further down the line, something interesting starts to happen. We focus on the progress in their move programme, the recovery focus and we back away from the scales! The results happen and I don't just mean the number on the scales. I mean the learning to give themselves time again, the realisation that they don't need to be sweating to be having a good workout, that they actually enjoy the exercise programme, and begin to want more and that they can eat food with no restrictions, just balance.

But the real magic is the self-confidence, the pride, the emotion, that internal voice that starts to change how it speaks to you.

Then your new found strength leads to life changing events such as coming off antidepressant medication, being the strongest yet even with ongoing osteoarthritis, lifting more than your bodyweight after being told you should "never lift heavy again" following a triple prolapse. Ditching the scales for good after 40 years of diets and negativity.

My business is called EMPOWER for a very clear reason. That is exactly what we do. That doesn't mean we all want to have the same gravitational pull on earth, wear the same clothes size, be scared of being bulky ..... be delicate?!

It's different for each of my clients but there is always a common ground. We are all going through a bloody challenging time, where we MUST give ourselves some of that time. We must prioritise physical strength to gain mental strength too.

With that comes true EMPOWERMENT

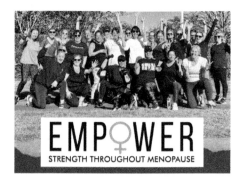

Scan the QR code to book your complimentary 20 minute consultation and enjoy 10% off any EMPOWER coaching programmes by quoting this book.

Notes:

To get started with my strength moves , I just need two 20 minute slots!

Where could I find these?

CHAPTER THIRTY NINE
Stress and Menopause
by Michaela Newsom

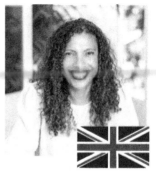

Bio: Michaela is a Registered Nutritional Therapist and a menopause expert who helps midlife women thrive through menopause. Michaela uses the latest scientific research alongside functional and genetic tests to understand the underlying functional imbalances that are causing your symptoms and then creates a foolproof, personalised plan based on your individual biochemistry designed to make you look and feel your best.

Business: Michaela Newsom – The Menopause Nutritionist
Website: www.michaelanewsom.co.uk
Instagram: @michaelanewsom

The life of the perimenopausal woman has never been more stressful. She has to perform numerous roles, wife, friend, mother, caregiver and career woman along with the expectation that she can have it all whilst looking like she did in her 20's. Research has shown that women suffer significantly higher levels of stress than men between the ages of 25 and 54. This is a particular issue for women at this age, as studies have shown that chronic stress can cause hormone levels to tank and can change the structure of the brain leading to brain shrinkage, memory loss and brain fog.

Why is this relevant? Well, although menopause is triggered by a decline in ovarian hormones, it all starts in the brain. More specifically, in a gland called the hypothalamus. The hypothalamus is where the signal to the ovaries originates and under chronic stress this signal is disrupted and can have a significant impact on the symptoms experienced during perimenopause.

When the brain senses danger, the 'fight or flight' stress response is activated. This response is an evolutionary survival mechanism, honed over millions of years and it prepares the body to confront or flee from danger.

Cortisol, the stress hormone, is released from the adrenal glands to prime the body for a "fight or flight" reaction. This involves increasing blood sugar levels to provide the muscles with energy to run or fight, increasing blood pressure to increase the delivery of nutrients and oxygen to the muscles and brain as well as switching off functions that are not immediately required such as digestion, the immune system and reproduction (let's face it, sex drive is not a priority when your life is in danger). By doing this, all available energy is diverted to survival mechanisms.

While short-term stress can be adaptive, chronic stress which is prolonged and unresolved can have detrimental effects on health. Unrelenting stress can change the outcome from protective to harmful.

This stress response evolved to help us respond to dangers such as sabre-toothed tigers. In these scenarios, once the danger passed, stress hormones returned to normal levels. However, in the modern world, this alarm system never turns off and we are exposed to chronic, unrelenting stress. The body cannot tell the difference between real, actual physical danger that needs a response or *perceived* danger. In today's world, we are stuck in a state of hypervigilance, the result of being available 24/7. We are constantly bombarded by social media, global news headlines, emails, financial worries, caring for ageing parents alongside young children, and the things that keep you up at night like climate or health disasters.

Stress can come in the form of physical stress (illness, trauma, accident, surgery), emotional stress (grief, anger, bereavement, insecurity, depression, overwhelm), dietary stress (caffeine, sugar, omega-6 fat overload, allergenic foods, nutrient deficiencies, food additives), medications (proton pump inhibitors, anti-inflammatory medications, the oral contraceptive pill, statins).

Menopause itself is a stress on the body and when combined with these external stressors it can increase the number and severity of symptoms.

By default, cortisol is produced in a diurnal pattern in which it is high in the morning, peaking around an hour after you get up (this is called the cortisol awakening response and gives us energy and get up and go in the morning) and then falls throughout the day to be low at night when cellular repair and healing happen. When stress is ongoing, this pattern can become disrupted leading to wider hormonal chaos.

Cortisol is the alpha hormone and rules over other hormones. It has an inhibitory effect on the production of some hormones such as oestrogen, progesterone, thyroid, growth hormone, melatonin but has a stimulatory effect on others, such as DHEA, testosterone.

The production of sex hormones starts in the hypothalamus where a hormone called gonadotropin hormone-releasing hormone (GnRH) is released. This hormone tells another gland in the brain, the pituitary, to produce luteinising hormone (LH) and follicle stimulating hormone (FSH). GnRH is released in pulses and the frequency of these pulses determines whether the pituitary releases LH or FSH. Cortisol changes the pulse rhythm of GnRH and reduces progesterone production, disrupting the delicate balance of oestrogen and progesterone, leading to unopposed oestrogen. This can cause disruption to the menstrual cycle with heavier periods, sore breasts, headaches, bloating and an increase in anxiety.

Another way cortisol can reduce levels of progesterone is by lowering thyroid hormone. Thyroid hormone is needed for a healthy menstrual cycle. Cortisol can block the signal to the thyroid gland to produce thyroid hormone leading to low thyroid hormone, which can result in a short luteal phase and lower progesterone increasing symptoms of low progesterone such as insomnia and anxiety. In addition, many symptoms of hypothyroidism are the same as menopause symptoms and so can make things much worse. Weight gain, constipation, fatigue, depression, brain fog, muscle aches and cramps are all signs of a struggling thyroid.

Melatonin is another hormone that is impacted by cortisol. Melatonin and cortisol are opposing hormones. When cortisol is high, melatonin is low. When cortisol is low, melatonin rises. This is why we get a rise in melatonin in the evening which triggers the onset of sleep. When cortisol is dysregulated and higher in the evening than it should be, it can make it difficult to fall asleep. Melatonin is also a powerful antioxidant and is essential for supporting the repair and healing overnight. This disruption to our natural biorhythms and circadian rhythm can affect sleep and cause fatigue, aches and pains.

As well as hormones, chronic stress impacts neurotransmitters which can exacerbate the neurological symptoms experienced in menopause. The downregulation of serotonin impacts mood and our ability to regulate our temperature which can exacerbate hot flashes. The suppression of dopamine can lead to a lack of motivation and drive whilst the loss of progesterone can reduce the activity of GABA which is the calming neurotransmitter leading to irritability, anxiety and insomnia.

As you can see, dysregulated cortisol can lead to multiple hormonal and neurotransmitter imbalances that can exacerbate the effects of perimenopause. For a smoother transition through perimenopause and into menopause, it is crucial to incorporate habits and routines that build resilience and reduce stress.

Here are fourteen ways to build resilience to stress and reduce cortisol;

1. Change the way that you perceive stress and respond to triggers – reframing can be a useful exercise to help you change the way you perceive a situation.

For example, "I'm stuck in traffic" when reframed becomes "I can use this time to listen to a podcast or enjoy some music". Or "I can't get everything done" can be reframed to "I'm prioritising tasks based on their importance and impact".

2. Breathwork – deep slow breathing activates the parasympathetic nervous system and helps us to calm down and reduce cortisol.

3. Yoga – the slow movements and focused breathing in yoga helps to activate the parasympathetic nervous system and has a calming effect on the body.

4. Meditation – is a way of calming the mind which decreases stress and stress hormones.

5. Exercise – research has shown that exercise can reduce cortisol levels and help reduce menopause symptoms.

6. Balanced diet – a poor diet with high sugar, inflammatory foods is a major stressor on the body. Poor blood sugar stability causes the body to balance blood sugar by releasing cortisol. To keep blood sugar balanced, avoid sugary foods, eat protein with each meal and do not skip meals.

7. Re-establishing circadian rhythm – Our circadian rhythm (including cortisol production) is dictated by the daylight cycles. Daylight triggers an increase in cortisol production whilst darkness switches of cortisol and switches on melatonin production. Exposing your eyes to outdoor daylight within 30 minutes of waking and avoiding blue light in the evenings will help to mimic our natural light-dark cycle.

8. Forest bathing or Shinrin-yoku is an ancient Japanese relaxation technique. Research has shown leisurely walks in the forest reduce cortisol levels by up to 12%.

9. Stimulate oxytocin – also known as the love or bonding hormone, oxytocin is the one hormone that can switch off cortisol. It is impossible to be stressed and relaxed at the same time. Oxytocin can be boosted with hugs, laughter, spending time with loved ones, stroking a pet or sex.

10. Prioritise me time – it's not a luxury to spend time doing something just for you. Take up a hobby or something that you enjoy doing to avoid.

11. Reading – the University of Sussex conducted a 2009 study that found that reading can reduce stress by up to 68%.

12. Massage – research shows that a one hour massage not only lowers cortisol but also increases serotonin which can relieve low mood and feelings of depression.

13. Grounding – walk barefoot on grass or sand. Free electrons in the earth flow into your body.

14. Build your tribe – the female response to stress is called tend and befriend. Women tend to band together and form tight friendships which from an evolutionary perspective enabled them to share resources. However, today women are often isolated, living miles from family and friends. Build a tribe with whom you can talk, vent, laugh and cry.

Menopause is inevitable but suffering isn't, so if you want to thrive through menopause book a call with Michaela and take the first step to feeling like you again.

Notes:

CHAPTER FORTY
Toxic Positivity in
Midlife: The Dark side
of Eternal Optimism
by Suzanne Laurie

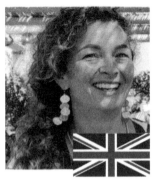

Bio: Suzanne is a midlife/menopause coach with a special interest in emotional and binge eating. She helps women navigate a healthy menopause, find food freedom and build body confidence. Suzanne has over 20 years experience as a wellness professional and educator, with qualifications in Nutritional Therapy (BSc. Hons), Positive Pyschology (MSc) and coaching .

Business: Mother Flushing Midlife
Website: www.motherflushingmidlife.com

Caveat: There will be no #goodvibesonly in this chapter - all vibes are acknowledged and welcome. We are human, we have feelings and I want you to get them out there! And as many of you may be knee deep in perimenopause those feelings are probably BIG hormone driven ones, which are probably not of the warm and fuzzy kind. These can feel uncomfortable, but they are also totally normal so ignoring them or hiding them away just leads to frustration, guilt and shame. In short, it's 'toxic positivity' and good things rarely come from a toxic start.

What is toxic positivity?

'Toxic Positivity' describes a disproportionate focus on life's positives while underplaying or ignoring negative emotions and circumstances. It's that idea of #goodvibesonly and the notion that we should ALWAYS be happy and optimistic as things 'could be worse'. I don't know about you but for me, perimenopause, and midlife in general, have certainly not been all rainbows and butterflies. In fact, I have days where I'm scraping the bottom of a very big barrel of negative to find any positivity at all - and I am known for my optimism.

But grinning and bearing things does not make midlife any easier to navigate – hot flushes are not fun. Mood swings and crippling anxiety...not so much either. Of course, there is nothing wrong with looking on the bright side and reminding ourselves of the good things in life during those darker days, but that has to be authentic. Simply ignoring challenges and the anger, frustration, sadness and confusion they invariably bring does not make them go away – in fact, it creates the perfect environment for them to fester and grow.

Being optimistic and positive doesn't involve pushing feelings aside and hoping for the best - it is knowing that whatever you are facing, you will get through it and there are many positive things ahead. But to do this we need acknowledge that all feelings are important and provide vital information about what is working or not working in our lives, and areas that might need our attention. They need accepting and working through before we can genuinely shift focus, otherwise they simply reappear at a later date, bigger, bolder and usually more destructive!

Examples of Toxic Positivity

- Not being honest with ourselves or others about the positives and negatives in life. Presenting only a carefully curated version of your reality to the outside World.
- Hiding what you really feel both from yourself and others.
- Dismissing, and feeling guilty for having, 'negative' emotions.
- Minimising other people's experiences with comments like 'everything happens for a reason', 'it's better not to dwell on things' or 'I'm sure it will all work out'. No judgement – we all do it, but in reality this is about minimising your own discomfort around their feelings rather than helping them process and move forward.
- Declaring 'it could be worse' or 'it's probably not as bad as you think' about someone's circumstances, which just inadvertently shames them for feeling bad.

Consequences of Toxic Positivity

The thing about toxic positivity is we all engage in it, often unconsciously. But here's why it's important we try to recognise when we are inadvertently tipping to toxicity scale.

- **We cannot selectively numb emotions:** If we numb the negative then we start to dull the positive feelings too.
- **Becoming disconnected from reality:** When you focus solely on the positives in life you are not acknowledging the full picture, which hinders your ability to make informed decisions and choices.
- **Invalidating important feelings:** Dismissing uncomfortable emotions (yours or those of others), diminishes their significance and can lead to guilt and shame. You might question your emotional experiences and deny yourself (or others) the opportunity for much needed support.
- **It becomes a false coping mechanism:** Instead of taking action to change a situation, you adapt and soldier on, keeping yourself stuck and fostering a sense of false powerlessness.
- **Avoidance and resistance:** Toxic positivity often serves as a tool for avoiding and resisting negative experiences. However, what we resist persists. By refusing to acknowledge the negatives, they only grow larger, perpetuating the cycle of avoidance.
- **Limited personal growth:** By disregarding the challenges and lessons that come with negative experiences, toxic positivity inhibits personal growth and development. True growth can only occur when we embrace and learn from all aspects of our lives.

Toxic Positivity in Midlife

Midlife can be like a perfect storm for some women, with

many challenges and changes (ageing, children leaving home, family illnesses and shifts etc) emerging just as our hormones go haywire. Whilst maintaining an unwaveringly positive attitude might seem appealing and noble, frankly – it's just a bad idea. Not just for you, but for other women experiencing the same issues, and for the next generations of women who will invariably go through the same struggles. We cannot and should not dismiss and invalidate the complex emotions and physical changes that women in this age group experience. The hormonal fluctuations and societal pressures are real and associated feelings of uncertainty, frustration, anger and self-doubt are normal. Soldiering on with a 'nothing to see here' attitude creates unrealistic expectations for all women, and means we also miss the many light and beautiful moments in our lives. We feel isolated, guilty and ashamed for being 'the only one' struggling. So, they then mask their genuine feelings, potentially exacerbating mental health struggles and making it harder to seek appropriate support – when research shows that community and support are incredibly important factors in reducing symptoms during the menopausal transition.

Embracing a more balanced approach that acknowledges both the ups and downs, highs and lows and potential roller coaster of midlife allows for dialogue. Dialogue supports understanding and change. It helps individuals, organisations and communities develop strategies to support midlife women in a healthier and more holistic way. It fosters genuine self-acceptance and emotional well-being during this transformative life stage. And let's face it, letting rip with those emotions just feels good. Better out than in!

Practicing Healthy Positivity

Healthy positivity involves authenticity. You can still be grateful for many things in your life (and you absolutely should be) whilst giving yourself, and others, the opportunity to acknowledge and navigate more challenging moments.

Here's how:

- **Seek supportive connections:** Surround yourself with a support network who understand and validate your experiences. Share your journey with trusted friends, family members, or seek professional guidance when needed. Engaging in open conversations can provide comfort, empathy, and a sense of belonging. It is also a fast track to reducing guilt and shame.

- **Practice self-compassion:** Be gentle and compassionate with yourself during moments of emotional distress. Recognise that negative emotions are normal. Treat yourself with kindness, offering yourself the support and understanding you would undoubtably offer a friend.

- **Cultivate emotional awareness:** Take time to check in with yourself, identifying and reflecting on your emotions. Acknowledge both positive and negative feelings without judgment. A feelings wheel (see below) is a handy tool to help you explore more subtle emotions hiding beneath the big and obvious ones such as anger, sadness and happiness.

- **Embrace authenticity:** Allow yourself to experience the full range of emotions. Savour moments of joy, but also acknowledge the challenges and lessons learned from difficult experiences. This balanced approach cultivates authenticity and emotional resilience. Understand that growth and personal development are dependent on accepting and navigating the ups and downs of life.

- **Journaling for emotional processing:** Consider regular journaling to process and explore your emotions. Set a timer for 20 minutes and write freely (without judgement), expressing all thoughts and feelings that come to mind in that time. This practice helps you gain clarity and understanding.

- **Have a social media cull:** Look at what your engaging with on social media and think about how it impacts your mood and mental health. Do some accounts make you feel inadequate? Unfollow. Do they contain a lot of trigger points for you e.g. body image issues? Unfollow. You get the picture.

The Feelings Wheel

Rejected · Helpless · Overwhelmed · Inadequate · Worthless · Excluded · Exposed · Betrayed · Disrespected · Violated · Jealous · Provoked · withdrawn · Apathetic · Pressured · Overwhelmed · Unfocused · Detestable · Dissapointed · Disgusted · Awful · Tired · Stressed · Busy · Bored · Distant · Aggressive · Hateful · Bitter · Humiliated · Let down · Threatened · Rejected · Weak · Insecure · Anxious · Scared

Victimised · Powerless · Ashamed · Empty · Disappointed · Peaceful · Relaxed · Sentimental · Content · Optimistic · Accepting · Satisfied · Amused · Enthusiastic · Pleasure · Excited · Passion · Cheerful · Fun · Joy · Bliss · Glee · Jolly · Comfort · Present · Focused · Trusting · Mellow · Relief · Hurt · Depressed · Guilty · Despair · Vulnerable · Lonely

Sad · Fear · Anger · Bad · Happy · Calm

@motherflushingmidlife

I say this with love, but ladies there is no award for martyrdom. It gets us nowhere and it breaks many of us along the way. I get it, as at times I've been guilty of some serious toxic positivity and undoubtably there will be more to come. Being honest about our feelings requires vulnerability, showing our darker side, which is incredibly uncomfortable.

But as midlife badass Brené Brown[1] states 'you either walk inside your story and own it or you stand outside your story and hustle for your worthiness'.

In other words – dare to be your true self. Know your value and stand with your messy emotions and struggles. Show other midlife women the highs, lows and everything in between, because it will help them and it will help you.

[1] https://brenebrown.com/

If you're ready to dive in, dig deep, shake off that comfort zone and step into a new way of approaching midlife and your relationship with food sign up to my newsletter via the QR code

Notes:

CHAPTER FORTY ONE
The Power of Tracking
by Emily Barclay

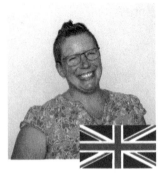

Bio: Emily, aka the peri-godmother, set up the perimenopause hub after over 3 years of feeling lost due to not understanding what was going on in her body. She now supports women through this life stage and provides corporate menopause education. Emily lives in Norfolk, UK, with her partner and too many dogs.

Business: Perimenopause Hub
Website: Perimenopausehub.com

Tracking your cycle unleashes your superpower!

For women, the menstrual cycle is a great tool to understand how they will feel and when. Our body is constantly giving us information, and if we track, we will quickly learn what to expect when.

If you start tracking when your cycle is regular, you will be in a much stronger position to explain what is wrong should you wish to see the doctor about any menstrual issues. And you don't need to have a period to track - if your birth control means you don't get a monthly bleed, don't panic, you can still track.

So what are you tracking? Well, firstly we need to look at the stages of the cycle and what signs your body might give you in each stage.

Menstrual phase

This runs from day one of the cycle. It is when you have your period. The average period lasts 3-7 days. If your period lasts longer than 10 days, it is worth getting checked by your Dr. You may experience bloating, cramps, fatigue and diarrhoea.

Follicular phase

This also starts on day one of the cycle, and runs until ovulation. During this time your body releases follicle stimulating hormone (FSH) to make the ovaries produce eggs. This phase lasts roughly 14 -16 days. Once the period is over, this is the time when you are likely to feel pretty good.

Ovulation

This is the time when an egg is released. It is the time when you are most likely to get pregnant. Ovulation lasts just 24 hours, and in this time you may notice you have higher libido. Your basal body temperature will be slightly higher from ovulation until the end of the cycle. You will get a discharge that has the consistency of egg whites, and you may notice some abdominal pain.

Luteal phase

This is the time when your body is doing what it can to protect a fertilised egg. The egg that was released at ovulation becomes the corpus luteum and releases hormones (primarily progesterone) to cause the womb lining to thicken. If you are not pregnant, then the corpus luteum is reabsorbed, causing oestrogen and progesterone to dip, which can lead to PMS. The luteal phase lasts 11–17 days (average is 14 days) so if you track ovulation, you will know more or less when to expect your next period.

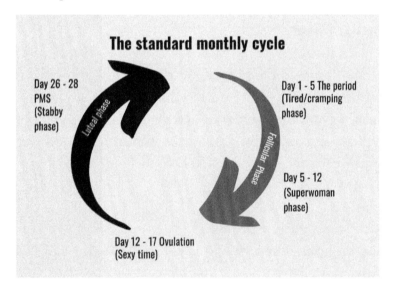

If you don't have a regular period, you can still track your cycle by looking at mucus, taking your temperature first thing every morning (before you move), noticing mood changes, observing sleep patterns, and making note of any food cravings.

Even if you are on hormonal birth control, there will be clues to tell you where you are in the cycle. Given that the majority of women are on some type of birth control it can be hard to identify where you are in your cycle. So I'm going to break down the different types and how they might impact you.

Combined pill

This contains oestrogen and progesterone, and aims to keep your hormone levels steady for 3 weeks and then on your 4th you have a bleed, when you have a break from taking the pill.

The bleed that you have isn't because you ovulated and didn't get pregnant (which it would be on a normal cycle) but it is because you have a hormonal bleed because you didn't give your body the usual dose of hormones.

Mini pill

This is a progesterone-only pill which you take every day without a break. You may still have periods while taking it, but if taken correctly it is 99% effective at preventing pregnancy.

Implant

The implant provides a steady stream of progestogen into the body which works to suppress ovulation and also to make the uterus a hostile environment for a foetus. Some women find they experience a light bleed with the implant, but many don't.

IUD

There are two different types of IUD (intrauterine device, otherwise known as a coil) – hormonal ones, such as Mirena, and non hormonal, such as the copper coil.

The hormonal coils release a low dose of progestogen into the uterus to thicken the mucus, making it harder for sperm to fertilise an egg, and to thin the uterine lining to ensure a pregnancy can't take hold. Women with the hormonal coil may still ovulate some months.

The copper coil, rather than releasing progestogen releases copper, which thickens uterine mucus making it hard for sperm to fertilise an egg. A woman's cycle will be unaffected.

Depo injection

This injection of the hormone progestogen suppresses ovulation to prevent an egg being released each month. It also thickens cervical mucus to stop sperm reaching the uterus.

Hysterectomy

If the reason you don't have a period is because you have had a hysterectomy, then so long as you still have your ovaries you will experience a cycle until you reach menopause as the ovaries will still be producing eggs. You may notice ovulation pain mid cycle, and this will be roughly 2 weeks before your period would be due.

What should you track?

In short, whatever you feel you need to. What do I mean by that? Well, given that we are all different, we all experience things slightly differently, we are all inconvenienced by different things, it makes sense that we would track the things that are right for us.

Personally, I now track bleed, pain, mood, sleep, energy levels, exercise and anything I feel needs noting on a particular day. But in the past I have tracked appetite, stress levels, response to stress, shortness of temper, and so on.

If you think about the symptoms you are experiencing, I would suggest starting with tracking the ones that impact you the most. I would also suggest you track exercise and whether any foodstuffs are having an impact on the severity of your symptoms. This doesn't need to be an all consuming task, it doesn't need to become like the obsessive food tracking one does when dieting, it can be more about noticing things throughout the cycle and noting them down with a view to comparing back at the same time in the next cycle.

After 3 months or so, you will likely have a much better idea of what your body is asking for at different stages in your cycle. You'll know when it wants you to slow down, when you can take on the world, when you want to eat non stop, when you'll sleep well and when your sleep may be more disturbed; and so much more. Your body holds the key to understanding and taking back control of your perimenopause.

So what is the benefit to tracking?

Well, it's being forewarned. No more surprise periods, no more being angry or feeling low and not understanding why until your period turns up a few days later. And once you get tracking you'll start to notice the times in your cycle when you have the most energy and the times when you are best off staying home. Armed with all this information you'll be in a much stronger position to know when you're going to ace the presentation at work and when you're best off declining social invites; when your partner and family will enjoy your company and when they'd do well to keep away from you. Tracking will also enable you to see that actually things aren't awful every single day, however much it may feel as though they are.

And once you have got to grips with this amazing superpower, you can start to talk to those around you and alert them to what to expect when. Your partner might want to know when you're ovulating so they can get some action, they might also want to know when the PMS phase (aka the stabby phase) is coming so they don't breathe too noisily in your general direction.

As you head into perimenopause, speaking to your partner and explaining what is going on becomes all the more important. It can be very easy to start to think that you're going crazy and that you must be imagining all the symptoms you are experiencing, but once you have a clear pattern linked to your cycle you find yourself back in control of what is happening, and it becomes very clear that you aren't imagining it – your symptoms are very real, even if some of them only happen once a month.

You may find your libido goes AWOL. Your partner may take umbrage at this, and start to believe you no longer fancy or love them. This is simply not the case (I mean it might be, but let's not go there right now!), rather your hormones are doing the conga and sex is the last thing they want. If you identify that you have a time in your cycle when you do fancy getting amorous, let your partner know. Make a date of it. Keep communicating. And if sex starts to be painful, which it does for many women as their oestrogen levels decline, please please seek help from your doctor – "relaxing with a glass of wine" isn't the answer here.

Many women find that among the first things they experience in perimenopause are some of the psychological symptoms including anxiety and low mood. If you have previously been a very confident upbeat person, these can come as a huge shock for you and for those around you. Keep talking to your partner and/or family. Explain how you are feeling. Also speak to your doctor - take the data from your cycle tracking to show that these mood changes are hormonal.

Can your loved ones help?

Yes, absolutely, but you may need to be the one to initiate the conversation. Research shows that talking side by side rather than face to face is better for men, in particular, to take more serious conversations on board, so you may find that rather that sitting down at a table to talk this stuff through, you will have more success if you chat in the car, on a walk, on a bike ride - anything where you are not looking directly at each other.

And show them any articles you find, show them this book, encourage them to learn about this life stage with you. If you can try to view this as the adventure it is, you will likely find you have an easier time, even if you experience the exact same symptoms as someone else.

My personal experience

In my early perimenopause days, before I knew why things were changing, I decided to start tracking what was going on. I downloaded a period tracking app onto my phone and set about making note of how I felt each day. Once I had enough data, I tried to export it to see any patterns, but there wasn't an export option so I painstakingly put each day's data into a spreadsheet so I could look at any patterns. It was worth it - this information showed me that my periods were all over the place, that my energy levels did vary with certain times in my cycle, that all these things were hormonal. In many ways it was a relief, although it was frustrating to have had to pull out all the data, rather than just being able to analyse it in the app!

With hindsight, I wish I had tracked my cycle, my moods, my energy levels and so on since my early 20s. I would have been so much better equipped to know when I would be epic and when I would need to be a bit more kind to myself.

I learnt that for me, the last week of my cycle is when I am lethargic. There is usually one day in that week when I have amazing focus for repetitive computer tasks, but I am best not doing too much physical activity. It is the week that I can get my accounts done without it feeling like a chore, but when the idea of a run is out of the question.

On the flip side, the few days around ovulation are when I can take on the world. I have energy, clarity of mind, fluency of language. On these days I can exercise more, I can liaise with people, I do some of my best work.

I've teamed up with the lovely people at Stella App, where not only can you track to your heart's content, you can also access doctors and get HRT prescriptions. Use the code HUB23 for £5 off per month for your first three months.

☆

Notes:

What are the top 5 things you would like to track? Think about the peri symptoms that are affecting you the most.

How would you like to track? Do you prefer paper or an app?

Get tracking!

Knowledge is power

CHAPTER FORTY TWO
Perimenopause &
Unresolved Trauma -
The Two Are Connected
by Nic Pendregaust

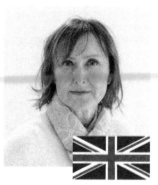

Bio: Helping peri-menopausal HR leaders feel lighter, brighter and in control and lead the way at work and at home. Nic is a qualified therapist with a counselling, coaching and hypnotherapy toolkit.

Business: Clarity Kent
Website: clarity-kent.co.uk

"Trauma is not what happens to you, it is what happens inside you as a result of what happens to you" Gabor Matte.

Unresolved Big or Little 'T' trauma can impact us in midlife. Perimenopause can be a difficult time for any woman due to hormonal fluctuations and midlife changes. 'Midlife' change can be many different things – challenging relationships with parents, siblings, career experiences that haven't sat well with you over the years, 'empty nest' syndrome, as children move out of home into their new place or go off to uni, grief and loss that you haven't processed – this can be losing a loved one or a concept coined by Julia Samuel 'living loss' that could be about loss of identity, health, purpose, confidence, self-esteem and/or relationship(s). So, any unresolved past issues can resurface, for us in our 'midlife'. And they do, don't they?

As ladies who have experienced trauma – in childhood, abusive relationships or PTSD, this sensitive time of life can reopen old, unresolved wounds, resulting in symptoms such as anxiety, depression, or panic attacks. Even hot flushes and night sweats can be exacerbated.

These things can continue to trigger us, if not fully looked at, understood and processed. We can go down the 'ostrich syndrome' route and suppress them or look to explore these unresolved past issues. If we choose not to recognise and deal with any unresolved issues & past trauma, we risk that they will hold us back in both our present and future. And you don't want that for yourself, do you?

We associate trauma and PTSD with the military or survivors of terrible disasters and the like. However, what we now know is that things such as childhood trauma and abusive relationships have the same effect on our nervous system. The person who experiences this can indirectly become conditioned to living in fight or flight mode – constant hyperarousal. It becomes a default setting in their nervous system. Dysregulation of our nervous system and the effect on our mental health can make our menopause symptoms more significant and severe. And entirely reasonable too, to experience delayed on-set PTSD, post pandemic.

Trauma impacts our bodies. Traumatic stress leads to a range of physical issues: in the brain, in the major organs of our body, in our immune system, in the stress response system itself.

Unresolved trauma is the greatest threat to our physical health.

Some stats, at a glance:
- 7.7x more like to suffer a stroke (Brass & Page, 1996)
- 62% increased risk of heart disease (Rich-Edwards et al, 2011)
- 2x more likely to develop chronic fatigue syndrome (Fuller-Thomson & Sulman, 2011)
- 65% higher risk of fibromyalgia (Fuller-Thomson & Sulman, 2011)
- 4.7x more likely to develop irritable bowel syndrome (Surdrea-Blaga, Baban & Dmuitrascu, 2012)

Bessel van der Kolk's definition of trauma is: 'an inescapably stressful event that overwhelms people's existing coping mechanisms'. We all have a different response to trauma. Trauma is often referred to as Big T or Little T trauma.

Big T we are talking those things that most people would consider traumatic, such as serious accidents, natural disasters, robbery, rape, violence, major surgeries, major life-threatening illness chronic or repetitive experiences (e.g., child abuse and neglect), war, combat and/or unexpected loss of a loved one. This may cause PTSD in some people, but not all.

A little T event is one experienced as traumatic at a personal level, it can include neglect, bullying, parental divorce, rejection, financial stress and/or break down of a relationship. Similarly, it can be experienced as catastrophic, life altering and distressing to our nervous system. Evoking too, feelings of powerless and low self-worth. Whereas big T trauma is commonly used to diagnose PTSD and complex PTSD, small T trauma can be overlooked. With big T we adopt active avoidance versus passive avoidance with small T (playing the experience down). Naming small T experiences as traumatic and validating them, can aid our recovery.

We hold emotional baggage & energy in our body – viscerally & somatically, hence this will show up physically and mentally for ourselves. As Bessel Van der Kolk says: 'The body keeps the score'. Whether our hormone fluctuations of menopause can trigger a trauma reoccurrence is still unknown and more research is needed, but for the women affected, the familiar lack of emotional control can cause anxiety, hyperarousal and vigilance and can disrupt their lives. Their radar is always up, and this is draining and tiring, creating stuckness and immobility.

Unresolved trauma can show up in our bodies with:

- Digestive issues
- Compromised immune system
- Chronic pain (Fibromyalgia, MS, Chronic fatigue)
- Hormonal changes
- Muscle & body tensions

- Limited movement
- Heart conditions
- Cancer
- Memory issues & trouble focusing
- Dizziness/vertigo
- Migraines & headaches
- High blood pressure
- Insomnia & sleep problems.

"Trauma comes back as a reaction, not a memory" – Bessel Van Der Kolk.

Unhealed trauma in childhood can be related to rejection, abandonment, betrayal & injustice. Not being seen or heard, having a parent deny your reality, having a parent who can't regulate their emotions, being told directly or indirectly that you can't show your emotions, having a parent that focused on appearance, and/or having a parent whose own emotions were dysregulated.

Unhealed childhood trauma can manifest in adulthood and potentially get triggered in midlife if not looked at - showing up as fixing others, people pleasing, codependency, needing external validation, hypervigilance, fear of abandonment, de-prioritising own needs, need for self-improvement, tolerating abusive behaviour, attracting narcissistic partners, difficulty in setting boundaries.

Trauma responses can manifest in various ways in our response to a threat. We can look at this in the context of the fight, flight, freeze or fawn response.

- **Fight:** workaholic, over-thinker, anxiety, panic, OCD, difficulty sitting still, perfectionism.
- **Flight:** angry outburst, controlling, bullying, narcissistic, explosive behaviour.
- **Freeze:** indecisive, stuck, dissociated, isolated, numb.
- **Fawn:** People pleasing, lack of identity, no boundaries, overwhelmed, co-dependence

Overlay hormonal changes and you can see there is a potential potent mix with unresolved trauma and perimenopause.

There are many ways to alleviate challenging symptoms both recognising that your old coping strategies no longer serve you (this could be - yet not limited to overeating, restricted eating, excessive drinking, excessive exercise).

- Taking time off work to prevent burnout
- Journalling
- Join support groups
- Reduce/stop alcohol & caffeine
- Good gut health
- Walks in nature
- Yoga/Qigong/stretching/breathwork
- Being creative -drawing, colouring, doodling & painting
- Somatic exercises
- Tapping (EFT)
- EMDR
- Therapy or counselling

- Support network – surround yourself with people who are supportive & empathetic

The earlier trauma is recognised, the quicker appropriate action can be taken to prevent symptoms lasting months or even years. HRT alone will not resolve the symptoms. Always speak to your health care provider for medical information. Yet therapy can – we need to 'feel to heal' and as Edith Eger says in her book, The Gift "The opposite of depression is expression. What comes out of you doesn't make you sick; what stays in there does." – Dr Edith Eger (Psychologist, Holocaust Survivor).

With my therapy, coaching and hypnotherapy experience and toolkit, I can help you to process and heal from any past unresolved traumas, which can trigger and destabilise us during our perimenopause, as well as support you with lifestyle modifications, and cognitive and behavioural ways to manage your psychological symptoms of perimenopause and menopause.

A note to anyone who needs to hear it...

We don't get over or move on from our trauma. We are forced to make space for it. We carry it. We learn to live with it. And sometimes, we thrive in spite of it.

If you feel that 1-1 therapeutic coaching with me is for you, book a free informal zoom coffee chat with me here: calendly.com/clarity-kent & let's start a conversation.

Notes:

Have you experienced Big 'T' and/or Little 'T' trauma?

What cues does your body give you, that may be linked to unresolved trauma?

Are your perimenopause symptoms being exacerbated by unresolved trauma?

What can you do differently to alleviate symptoms?

CHAPTER FORTY THREE
The Bits You Need to
Know About Your Bits
by Victoria Howell

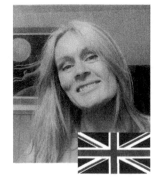

Bio: Hi, I'm Victoria. I graduated from the University of East Anglia in 2003 as a Registered Nurse Adult (RNA), I have worked both in primary and secondary care as a community nurse, practice nurse, CHC nurse assessor and senior clinical management. I'm also a trained coach. I trained further, and continue to develop, with the FSRH, PCWHF and British Menopause Society. I provide staff menopause clinics for the NHS and work for Holland and Barrett as a menopause nurse. I provide menopause workshops in the workplace, including general awareness, managers training and train menopause champions.

I am a co-founder of Women's Health Education Network Norfolk or WHENN, which was formed in 2022 with the aim of providing free education for healthcare professionals working in primary care we also hold both webinars and face-to-face events for the public.

Business: Victoria Howell Menopause Services
Website: www.victoriahowellmenopauseservices.com

Genitourinary Syndrome of Menopause (GSM)

The first thing you need to know about your "bits" is that they are not called "bits" at all! Nor are they called lady garden, noo noo, beaver, down there, or see you next Tuesday. If you were to speak to a registered healthcare professional, and say you have a sore noo noo, they will likely think you are talking about the Telly Tubbies Hoover, and advise you to see an electrician, get my point? Great, I am so glad we have cleared that up.

Now down to business, no not another analogy folks, the correct term for the outside genitalia of a female is called the vulva, the vulva itself is made up of several areas, we will go into that later. Where the vulva enters inside the body, this is called the vagina, again, made up of various components.

Please refer to the free vulval check guide (at the end of the chapter).

What's going on?

GSM or genitourinary syndrome of menopause can affect one or more organs in the pelvic cavity such as the vagina and bladder, it also affects the vulva. We have oestrogen receptors all over our bodies, doing amazing jobs at keeping us ticking along all tickety boo. Oestrogen is not just a component to enable pregnancy. Nor is it the only hormone involved in menstruation, you also need other hormones such as progesterone, they are a team.

Our very clever bodies rely on oestrogen for various roles and there are oestrogen receptors in many parts. While systemic HRT (so think patches, sprays, or gel) help with symptom control such as emotional, mental, and physical such as hot flushes, joint pain etc very little if any of that reaches the pelvic organs.

So, what are the symptoms of oestrogen deficiency in the pelvic organs? If you find yourself waking up during the night needing to wee, we call that nocturia, some wake up several times a night and of course that impacts sleep quality and energy levels, other symptoms include regular urinary tract infections, frequency, and urgency of the need to wee.

You can also experience symptoms which include a burning sensation in the vagina, friction during walking and/or intercourse, painful penetration due to decreased lubrication during sexual intercourse, irritation, itching and tissue frailty.

The Vulva
Knowing the correct names for your genitals is crucial whenever you require a GP appointment about any concerns. The external genitalia is the vulva, not to be confused with the vagina, which is inside your body. The vulva consists of folds and crevices, including the labia majora, labia minor, clitoral hood, clitoris, and entrance to the vagina (vestibule).

The Vagina
The vagina is the route from the vulva to the cervix and uterus. The lining of the vagina is plump, cushiony, and

moist, it naturally stretches to accommodate events such as birth or penetration (the stretchy part is called the ruggae). This contains naturally occurring lubrication, triggered by oestrogen. When oestrogen levels decline and plummet, the lining becomes thin, dry, and less elastic, therefore cannot stretch like before. Vaginal secretions called discharge change and become alkaline which can burn and excoriate the lining of the vagina. The sides of the vagina can rub together and cause pain during activities such as intercourse, having a smear test, riding a bike, walking, sitting or simply wearing a pair of jeans. This can cause sustained pain which results in low mood, pain, and misery.

The Bladder
What's the bladder got to do, got to do with it? See what I did there?

Well, rather a lot actually. The urethral sphincter acts as a door which opens from the bladder to release urine out of the body, and it closes once urination has stopped. When we have a lack of oestrogen that door can become a bit fluttery, especially if the pelvic floor muscles have become weak. Close to the urethral sphincter, there are lots of oestrogen receptors, which soak oestrogen in to enable that door to be either open or closed, not like a door blowing in the wind that allows rogue urine to escape.

Under-reported and under-diagnosed
Genitourinary syndrome of menopause is underreported and underdiagnosed and as a result, is therefore under-treated. A

very small percentage of women seek help circa 25% (Dr Heather Currie, WHC). The genitals are a private aspect of an individual's body and life. It can be excruciatingly embarrassing to talk about any noted issues of the vagina/vulva even to healthcare professionals. Please try not to worry. Our healthcare professionals are used to supporting people with all types of body functions and issues, so please know you will not be judged in any way whatsoever. The vulva, vagina and bladder are part of the body just like the back or head.

It is important to see a healthcare professional for any symptoms you experience, so they can help you. If you find it difficult to talk directly about burning, stinging, or itching of the vagina or vulva, you can take the infographic along with you, and point to where you may be having pain/discomfort etc, it will be a gentle way to approach the conversation.

Symptoms of oestrogen deficiency in the bladder, vagina, and vulva.

Urgency and/or frequency of urine. You may find yourself going for a wee just before leaving the house, we call that a "just in case" wee. You may find that you wear a panty liner at work in case you sneeze, for added protection against leaks and malodour.

Recurrent urinary tract infections can be due to a lack of oestrogen and pelvic floor dysfunction such as a cystocele, where the uterus is leaning down onto the bladder. This misshapes the bladder slightly therefore a small amount of residual urine can get left behind, leading to a urinary tract infection.

Itching of the vulva area including the mon pubis (the hairy section), perineum (between vulva and anus), vulva and inside the vagina is symptomatic of GSM. Other symptoms include 'being aware' of the vulva and/or vagina when going about your day-to-day lives. The pain of the vulva and vagina may also feature. Pain during penetrative sex is due to thin vaginal walls and shrinkage to the opening of the vagina. Symptoms such as burning in the vagina, reduced or absent sexual desire and arousal, reduced sexual pleasure and impaired orgasm. Another sign is a change in the odour of the vaginal secretions and vulval area.

I'm sure you have all heard of the gut microbiome, well did you know the vagina has its very own microbiome? As the PH changes from acid to alkaline the microbiome becomes unbalanced resulting in malodour and increased susceptibility to and frequency of infections.

Symptom checker

If you have any of these symptoms, do go and get checked by a healthcare professional within your GP surgery. Head over to look at the GSM symptom checker on the Menopause Support[1] website, listed in resources for more information.

[1] http://www.menopausesupport.co.uk/

Treatment options

GSM is what we term a chronic or long-term condition. So, what does that mean? Well, without continuous treatment it will return, it won't get better by doing nothing. This means that symptoms will progress and become even more painful and have a further detrimental impact on your day-to-day living.

Local oestrogen is available on prescription from your primary care prescriber such as a GP, Practice Nurse, or Nurse Practitioner. It's available in a variety of forms. Small tablets, pessaries, creams, or gels. When commencing local oestrogen, it is inserted into the vagina last thing at night for two weeks. Following that it is used twice weekly as a maintenance dose. If you have noted shrinkage and paling of the vulva you will notice how it re-plumps and regains a healthy colour demonstrating blood flow to the area.

Lubricants

There are a variety of lubricants on the market for you to choose from, there are so many that it can be difficult to know which to purchase. Tingling types of fruity flavours, while they may make everything slightly slip sliding away, are very short-term. Many of these contain glycerine, which helps things feel slippery for a short while, but it dries the delicate lining of the vagina and the vulva out longer term, so can have an adverse effect on what you try to achieve. Look for products that do not contain glycerine, YES[2] is a reputable

[2] http://www.yesyesyes.org/

428

brand and is available in most chemists, online and on prescription. Sutil[3] is another excellent brand, again this one does not contain glycerine and nurtures the vaginal mucosa.

Vaginal Moisturiser

YES, vaginal moisturiser, again available in chemists, online and on prescription. Sutil is available to purchase online and although is primarily a lubricant the Rich version provides long-term vaginal moisturisation and many women who cannot take local oestrogen use Sutil as a preferred moisturiser.

Vaginal moisturiser can be used in addition to local oestrogen after showers or on non-local-oestrogen days.

The Jo Divine[4] website sells Sutil lubrication and provides fact sheets on sexual and vaginal health.

The Women's Health Concern[5] website is the public arm of the British Menopause Society therefore all fact sheets are evidence based written by medical menopause specialists in collaboration with the Medical Advisory Council of the British Menopause Society.

So peeps, no more feeling shame about talking about your vulva, vagina or perineum, hold your heads high and shout it loud and proud ●

[3] http://www.sutillube.com/
[4] http://www.jodivine.com/
[5] http://www.womens-health-concern.org/

To grab your free vulval check guide and symptom checker, or just to have a wander around my website, just scan the QR code:

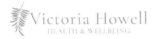

Victoria Howell
HEALTH & WELLBEING

Vulva Check Guide

We all know that we should check our breasts monthly. Well, did you know we should be checking our vulva monthly too?

Why? There are a variety of vulval skin conditions that can often get overlooked or mistaken for thrush or a urinary tract infection. Therefore, it is important to examine yourself to know your baseline and be aware of any changes. There are a variety of vulval and vaginal skin conditions such as: genitourinary syndrome of menopause (or vulvovaginal atrophy), lichen sclerosus, lichen planus, lichen simplex, vulval intraepithelial neoplasia (VIN), candida infection, psoriasis and vulval cancer.

Many women avoid talking to their health care professional about vulval issues because they are embarrassed. We need to normalise vulval and vaginal issues, so people do not feel embarrassed and can access the right care. This how to guide can help you on the right track.
The vulva is the external genitalia of a women, see diagram below.
The diagram right shows you the vulva in more detail. You need to be able to identify the different areas in the vulva, to enable the Dr to make a diagnosis. For example, if you say you have an itchy vagina, you may get a diagnosis of thrush, when you meant your vulva, when in fact it could be one of the skin issues listed. If you go and see your Dr to talk about your vagina or vulva, take a diagram with you so you can point to the area before being examined. You will also find it useful to take a mirror with you, so when the Dr refers to a certain part, you can see. This is particularly useful when being advised how to apply certain topical ointments.

To check your vulva, grab a mirror and make yourself comfortable.

- Site the mirror so you can see the reflection of your vulva.
- With a clean hand, gently prise open your labia major.
- You will now see the other areas that make up your vulva.
- Gently & carefully look around the labia major, labia minor, gently moving the vulval skin to see the clitoral hood, clitoris, urethral opening, and vestibule.
- While checking, pay attention to your perineum and anal area.

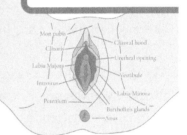

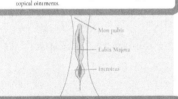

Physical signs you may have vulval/vaginal skin issues:

- Itching
- Burning
- Painful intercourse
- Post coital bleeding
- Bleeding from the vagina or vulva (non-period related)
- Burning when passing urine
- Becoming aware of your vagina when walking, sitting
- Painful sitting
- Urinary tract infection symptoms
- Getting up to wee during the night

Visual signs to look out for:

- Red patches
- Purple patches
- Raised white patches
- Splits
- Lump or wart like growth
- A mole that changes colour or shape
- Tears
- Blister
- ulcers
- Sores
- Crinkled, creased shiny looking skin
- Thinning and/or fusing of the labia major & labia minor
- Shrinking of the clitoris

Notes:

CHAPTER FORTY FOUR
Who am I now?
Reconnecting with you!
by Emma Roache

Bio: Emma Roache is an experienced coach who started her coaching journey in 2007 and has undertaken extensive coach specific training, alongside a BSc in Social Science with Criminology, and at the time of writing is studying towards a MSc in Psychology. However, the thing which makes Emma different is her life experience, having overcome numerous adversities including childhood trauma, abusive relationships and significant bereavements to name a few, Emma comes from a place of knowing, of deep empathy and is someone who walks beside you to empower you, with a coaching style which is based in science, and delivered with love! Outside of coaching Emma loves to travel, to swim in the North Sea even throughout the winter, and is a huge fan of Norwich City Football Club!

Helping You Be Happier
Website: www.emmaroache.com

'I promise you, selfcare is not selfish, it is essential, and you are important, and you deserve to live a full and happy life!'

Our identity changes as we go through life, however during perimenopause, it is quite typical that we begin to question everything, and one of the questions I hear from the women I work with is... who am I? Does that sound familiar to you?

Questions around who we are now come up for a number of reasons, which fundamentally come down to the fact that everything feels like it is changing and that we have no control over it and as a result can feel a little bit lost at sea.

Some examples of how we may feel at this time are:

- My body is changing, am I still who I thought I was?
- My moods and emotions are changing and feel unpredictable, I no longer feel like me...
- I feel sad, unmotivated, confused and I am worried I may never be happy again!
- I used to be fun and have fun, but I feel like I have lost my sparkle, my mojo, my drive...
- My children are leaving home, what is my purpose now?
- Now the children are leaving I am not sure I want to stay in my relationship...
- I am worried about my relationship now things are starting to change, I am more anxious, less tolerant, I don't know how to be in a relationship any longer.
- I should be married, have children, be settled by now and I feel like a failure...
- I seem to have lost 'me' along the way... my other roles (career, family commitments etc) felt more important and looking after me is selfish isn't it?

Firstly, I just want to add that some of these things are social norms which are projected onto us and are not the things we really feel deep inside, we may only feel this way because society says you should, and if that is the case then society can stuff their expectations! This is all about you and unhelpful social norms are just that. I only want you to consider things you genuinely feel for yourself, not the things society tells you that you should feel or be!

So when we start to notice we are feeling a bit lost, that we aren't quite sure who we are in this phase of our lives, we may start to notice we don't quite know how to navigate it, and that can feel unsettling and confusing.

The good news is there are things we can do to reconnect with ourselves and learn to love ourselves again, ways to discover who we are now and to choose who we would love to be in the future, who we are evolving into.

Sometimes just knowing we aren't alone is a comfort, so I promise you, even if you feel like it, you are not alone! I know this stage can feel incredibly lonely, we can feel like we are the only one going through this, that no one understands, that if we speak to people they will judge us, worry about us, or simply make us feel a little silly for feeling how we feel, but at the same time we are desperate for support, connection, understanding and to be able to find a way out of the way we feel.

Working with a trained professional like myself can be really helpful and some of us really need that external support to make sense of what is going on for us, to process what feels confusing, overwhelming and so on, but I understand that this isn't an option for everyone, so I will share some thoughts, ideas and tips to help you to start to navigate this tricky time and start to reconnect with you!

Ready? To start with we need to get the basics right. I know this sounds simple and easy to say, and it can feel tricky to do, to fit things in when we are super busy, or to commit to something new if we are feeling tired, stuck, and unmotivated. So I invite you to consider what you may be able to commit to right now, no matter how small or insignificant it may feel, I promise you that starting with small manageable goals and building upon them is way more successful than aiming for too much too quickly and then feeling like we have failed again, because big changes are hard and they don't come easily; small, steady and manageable is the way!

- The number one best thing you can do for your physical, mental, and emotional wellbeing is sleep and around 7-9 hours is what we are aiming for... I know, I know, sleep, or the lack of sleep is one of the peri symptoms many of us struggle with, but what we can do is rest. A good bedtime routine can help with this, reducing screen time, reading a book, having a relaxing cuppa, using relaxing essential oils or a warm bath or shower and so one, whatever works for you, what this does is sends signals to our brain that we are preparing for sleep, and we are choosing activities which rest our minds and our bodies. When I struggle to sleep, I use a meditation app, or play relaxing music, or count backwards from 10000, this gives our brain something to do which is enough to keep it from thinking about all the other things we are worried about, but not too much to keep us awake. Are you willing to try it?

- The next things are eating and drinking as healthily as we can, the fuel we give our bodies impacts how we feel, choosing healthier nourishing options is also an act of self-care, plus of course the things we love, but if we are honest we know the foods which don't agree with us and make us feel less good, but sometimes they're quicker to grab even though we know other options make us feel good inside!

- Find connection, whether that be with friends or loved ones, with nature, or with you... finding connection is an important element of our wellbeing and depending on our circumstances we will have different things which energise us, which helps us to recharge the batteries. For me spending time alone in nature, connecting with the world around me is something which really brings me joy, for you it may be catching up with a good friend or family member, or maybe starting a new hobby with others!

- Move your body! This can be whatever works for you, whether you go to the gym, swim, do yoga, go for a walk or a run, or put on your favourite tunes and dance around your house like no one is watching. Moving our body makes us feel good! And moving our body when we feel stuck, literally changes the way we think and feel!

By doing these things, or slowly building them in, we are starting to show ourselves love, care and attention, we are choosing to give ourselves time and permission to look after ourselves and show ourselves the love and consideration we often do for others. We start to feel more confident, more resilient, and more connected to ourselves.

When we do this, our perception of ourselves starts to shift, our mood lifts and we feel lighter, we realise we are important too. We are then more able to take time to take a step back and check in with how we are really feeling, what we are noticing in the world around us and what feels right for us now.

We start to get to know ourselves again; what we like, and importantly what we don't like. We reconnect with what we value, what we wish for and what we aspire to, we allow ourselves to dream! We reconnect with the things which light us up and make us shine, the things which give us a sense of purpose, and which form the parts of our identities which are important to us, the parts of us we thought we had lost. We even find and shape new parts of ourselves which are exciting too!

I invite you now to make a list of things which bring you joy, it can be anything, it can be a walk, being at the beach or in the woods, cooking, reading, sleeping, watching your favourite program, a long forgotten hobby, or something you have always wanted to try and so much more, the only important thing is that it means something to you and lights you up.

I promise you, selfcare is not selfish, it is essential, and you are important, and you deserve to live a full and happy life!

Now over to you, what are you willing or able to commit to?

Good luck! I believe in you, and I know this stuff works, it may feel slow at first, but in time you will start to notice and feel the benefit, if you have any questions, or concerns, wonder what it would be like to work with me, or simply want to
share with me you successes I would love to hear from you! And if you found this helpful, I send a weekly email too which you can sign up to via my website above. You've got this!

Journal prompts:

What are the things which bring me joy?

What are my dreams and aspirations?

What actions am I willing to commit to?

'Do or do not, there is no try!' Yoda

CHAPTER FORTY FIVE
Menopause at Work
by Emily Barclay

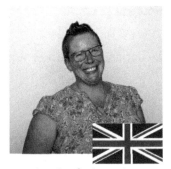

Bio: Emily is passionate about ensuring nobody feels as lost in perimenopause as she did. She offers menopause education sessions for businesses, as well as advising on how companies can best support their staff "of a certain age". Emily lives in Norfolk, UK, with her partner and too many dogs.

Business: Talk Meno
Website: Talkmeno.com

We are the first generation who have not only been encouraged to "have it all", but more or less expected to; meaning we are the first generation where the vast majority of perimenopausal age women are in work, as well as juggling all the other life things that previous generations of women would have been dealing with. Somewhere along the line, the men of our generation didn't quite get the memo that if the women are to "have it all", they need to do more than just go to work.

In their 2019 research, the Chartered Institute of Personnel and Development (CIPD)[1] in the UK found that 59% of working women between the ages of 45 and 55 who are experiencing menopause symptoms say it has a negative impact on them at work. They found that nearly a third of women had taken sick leave because of their symptoms, with only a quarter of those taking sick leave feeling able to tell their manager the actual reason why they needed time away from work.

Unfortunately, the CIPD advice still focuses on hot flushes being the primary symptom that should be addressed, suggesting that women have access to a desk fan and are able to have more breathable uniform. These are great for those who struggle with hot flushes, but 25% of women don't experience them, and there are many many other symptoms that have a greater impact.

Those of us reading this book know there are **WAY** more symptoms than just hot flushes, indeed have probably learnt that if we are going to experience them, they'll come on as we get closer to menopause rather than earlier in perimenopause.

So what symptoms might affect us in the workplace?
- Anxiety
- Insomnia
- Fatigue
- Poor concentration
- Low mood

[1] https://www.cipd.org/uk/about/press-releases/menopause-at-work/

442

- Brain fog
- Dizziness
- Imposter syndrome
- Flooding periods
- Extreme period pains
- PMS
- Low mood

And many more. Having access to a desk fan won't help with any of those, sadly!

To create change, we need to be the change. We need to be not only the generation who "has it all", but the generation who talk about it all. Menopause has been taboo for far too long, it has been endured (or rather, women were put in asylums rather than anyone acknowledge their hormones were running amok) but never spoken about. Together, we can change that.

Elsewhere in this book you will find numerous ways to address different symptoms with lifestyle changes, supplements, medical intervention and much more; but while you're doing all the good stuff you may well still be struggling at work. Let's address how you can get your employer and colleagues on board to support you through your hormonal rollercoaster.

Colleagues
Your colleagues are the people who see you every day. They're the ones who pick up the slack when brain fog hits,

so we'll start with them.

However uncomfortable it might feel to talk about menopause, they will only be able to help you if you open the conversation. This bit is on you, I'm afraid! Time to find the communication style you're happy with.

- Do you have one colleague you are closer to in whom you can confide how you're feeling, and maybe ask them to have a quiet word with the others?
- Perhaps you'd feel more comfortable saying something in a small team meeting
- You might be an upfront "say it as it is" type
- Email may be your preference

Whatever your chosen route, start letting those around you know that things are a bit different right now. Focus on the primary couple of symptoms that are really affecting you, and ask your team for their help. Let's say your biggest workplace symptoms are poor memory and flooding periods, get into the habit of asking colleagues to email any requests to you, telling them you won't be able to action anything you don't have in writing; for the heavy periods, you don't need to go into the nitty gritty, but tell them that from time to time you will be going to the loo more often than usual, and that sadly it's beyond your control.

For those colleagues who choose to be unhelpful or unsupportive, kindly remind them that they make allowances when women are pregnant, and that your hormones are doing something similar, just minus the baby at the end. Remember, if people are consistently unsupportive, your HR department should be able to step in. I can't state enough how important talking about how you're doing will help you as well as those around you. It will feel uncomfortable initially, but it'll get easier – as with all things, if you take ownership of it, you retain control.

Employer
In an ideal world, your employer would have a menopause policy. In this same ideal world, they would have menopause marshals, just as they might have mental health first aiders. However, I know we don't live in an ideal world.

You are absolutely within your rights to request reasonable adaptations to help you thrive at work. These might include:
- Flexible working hours, including time to attend Dr appointments
- Sanitary products in the toilets
- The opportunity to work from home at certain times of the month
- Regular short breaks through the day
- A "breakout" area

And more.

Many workplaces now host menopause education sessions, which are a great opportunity for the topic to be discussed without it needing to be all about you. If you think it would be beneficial for your workplace to learn more, don't hesitate to get in touch with me – the joy of Zoom means we can very easily set this up, and what's great is that people can attend from anywhere and don't even need to take the terrifying step of walking into the meeting room to learn more.

As I have previously mentioned, we are the first generation talking about this, so don't be surprised or unduly put off if your employer doesn't yet have these things in place. Reframe it that you are helping future women. Don't forget, someone has to be first to do everything - might as well be you!

Ultimately it is in your employer's interests to keep you in the job, rather than have to go through the recruitment rigmarole, especially if you've been there a long time and are a valued staff member. Similarly, it is in their best interests to keep you working rather than signed off on long term sick leave. To be brutally honest, most employers don't want to deal with all the paperwork if they can avoid it!

You

We've looked at your colleagues and your employer, but the most important person in all this is you. What do you want? Do you want to stay in full time employment, or actually is perimenopause causing you to reevaluate your life? Maybe now is the time to go part time, to change jobs, to set up your own business. There is no right or wrong here. The only right or wrong is what is right or wrong for YOU.

If staying in your job is the right answer, consider what sort of colleague you have been until now, and whether this is still serving you - have you always been the person who picks up the slack and sorts everything? Maybe now you need to start setting some boundaries. Saying no can feel very daunting, but starting with something like "I don't have time today, I can help tomorrow" is a good way to begin to push back against those people who expect too much from you. Have you always been the super organised person who remembers everything, but now you find you've forgotten a few bits? Find some co-working apps that can help, use your reminders on your phone, write lists.

Ultimately, the menopause transition is going to happen, work is going to happen. Now is the time to establish what you need and to implement that.

Reach out if you need help and support. I run menopause education sessions for workplaces. I want every workplace to be menopause friendly.

Click on the QR code for more information about my menopause at work sessions:

Notes:

What are my biggest perimenopause-related struggles at work?

What adaptations would make these have less of an impact?

What is my preferred communication style around my peri symptoms?

Who should I contact for more support?

You deserve to feel comfortable at work

CHAPTER FORTY SIX
You are an Extraordinary Human. Body Acceptance: A Beginner's Guide.
by Emily Barclay

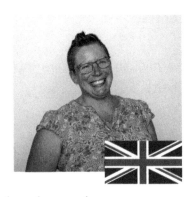

Bio: As well as being the peri godmother and a menopause educator, Emily is a personal trainer who focuses on helping women feel epic in the body they are in. In her ideal world, every woman would be able to see her inherent worth without the internal voice chipping in with negativity. Emily lives in Norfolk, UK, with her partner and too many dogs.

Your body is merely a vessel for your awesomeness as you journey through life.

Let me start by saying you are perfect exactly as you are. Even if you don't quite believe me just yet.

Just as our body changed through puberty, so it changes in perimenopause. For many of us this brings up all sorts of old feelings of being somehow in the "wrong" body. Being the "wrong" size or shape.

Add to this the constant societal noise about how being slim is somehow better, the fat-shaming that is inherent in the medical world, and the way larger bodies are portrayed in movies, and it's little surprise we can end up feeling distinctly ill at ease with our own body.

However... YOUR BODY IS EPIC.

Honestly, your body is epic. It is the amazing thing that houses all your wonderful personality, morals, kindness, humour and everything else. If you have had children, it has grown them. If you are sporty, it enables you to do that. If you are arty or crafty, yep it's your body that gets you doing that.

The number in your clothes label doesn't make you less kind, funny, generous, intelligent. It doesn't make you less of a friend. It doesn't make you a lesser person.

There is a movement called Body Confidence. I appreciate the sentiment. It'd be great if we could all be confident in our skinsuit. However, to go from disliking (nay, hating in some cases) what you see in the mirror or in photos to feeling confident is a bit of a reach for many of us. Let's aim for body acceptance.

What is body acceptance?

It is gently moving away from hating what your body looks like, what it represents for you, towards accepting it is a body like any other, and that it's yours and yours alone.

It is catching the negative thoughts before they consume you.

It is starting to be OK with taking up the space that you take up, rather than feeling you need to be smaller.

It is simply accepting that your body is doing a great job of housing all your epicness.

And how do I do that then?

Start small. Start with noticing the negative thoughts. Simply noticing them. Next time you look in the mirror and your internal voice says "Jeez you look godawful in that, you've really let yourself go, who'd ever love you" (yes, I know how brutal the inner voice can be), just observe it.

Then, while still looking in the mirror, look at a part of you that you like. Your eyes, maybe; your smile; your hair; hell, your fingernails! Remind yourself that underneath that skin is an amazing person.

Once you have started to notice these horrible thoughts, you can begin to counter them with facts about you.

Horrible thought:
- "Jeez, you look godawful"
- "Whatever possessed you to wear that?"

Possible counters:
- "I give the best hugs, without this body I couldn't do that"
- "I am a kind person, without this body, I wouldn't be able to share my kindness"
- "I am intelligent, without a body I wouldn't be able to do X, Y, Z clever things"

Diet culture and our relationship with our body

In the last few decades, the rise and rise of diet culture has meant it is very hard for us to be at peace with our body, as we are constantly being offered ways to "better" it. These messages come at us from the TV, the radio, magazines, social media, friends, family. The "slimmer is better" message is ubiquitous. And yet in countries where the diet message is strong, bodies are getting bigger!

In the case of certain illnesses, we are given the message that our body size is the issue. That we are at fault. We get told simply to eat less and move more. These messages are not helpful. They lead to people in larger bodies to avoid seeking medical help when it is needed, as they are so fearful they will be blamed for any ailment they have; so they don't go to the Dr until it is really serious[1].

If we could remove fatphobia from our medical system, I suspect we would see a marked reduction in these awful cases of larger people not seeking help until they are in dire need, which in turn would likely show a marked reduction in the

[1] https://www.ncbi.nlm.nih.gov/pmc/articles/PMC6565398/?fbclid=IwAR3ebhsrE2SKe-iLztNVmNvb7kwmlUc18A_9jLWq8_ow4nQD9UXaG47CJjM#:~:text=Fat%20shaming%20is%20also%20linked,and%20turn%20it%20on%20themselves

correlation of larger equalling less healthy.

This, obviously, is an issue at the other end of the scale, too. People slip through the net when they are very poorly but an acceptable BMI, as they are "fine".

The sooner we can move away from BMI as a mode of determining health the better. As an aside, did you know that BMI was created by a mathematician to find "the average man"[2]. The data used in that initial study was from European males. Immediately we can see that BMI was never intended as a health tool, nor was it inclusive of women, BAME people, and so on. Flawed? Yes. Widely used? Absolutely. A reason to hate yourself? Absolutely not. Please, from this moment on, don't let a mathematical study that didn't even include people with boobs define your self worth.

My body acceptance journey

Now, if you're reading this thinking "easy for you to say, Emily, bet you've always been one of those people who is happy with their body", you couldn't be further from the truth.

From a very young age, I thought I was "too big". Initially this was because my best friend when I was a child is petite, so even if I wasn't "too big", next to her I was taller, bigger, took up more room, and so on. While I didn't know how to acknowledge that feeling when I was 6, it has stuck with me

[2]https://www.ncbi.nlm.nih.gov/pmc/articles/PMC4890841/#:~:text=It%20was%20developed%20by%20Dr%20Quetelet%20in%20the%201800s.&text=In%201972%2C%20Keys%20et%20al,who%20were%20underweight%20or%20overweight.

for many years.

Moving forwards to puberty, I remember thinking that if I could just restrict what I ate I'd have the "perfect" body. I'd relentlessly scrutinise every part of myself, finding fault everywhere.

Through my 20s and 30s I veered dramatically between being a size I felt was "worthy" and being a "failure" when I inevitably re-gained the weight. I was so desperate to be an acceptable size that I tried endless diets, even considered those weight loss pills you see in the chemist.

The crazy thing is that when I now look back at photos from those years, I see an attractive woman who wasn't in any way fat. I also, however, see a woman who didn't quite know what her place in the world was, and felt that controlling her body size might help her to fit in better.

So, what changed?

My headspace changed. I finally became tired of hating myself for simply being a human in a body. I read an amazing book called Beyond Chocolate by Audrey and Sophie Boss, which helps people move away from diet culture and find peace with food.

I removed diety things from my social media, from my controllable world. I stopped complimenting others on their body size/shape, and started to focus on other things - a new haircut, the fact they look happy, a necklace, whatever.

I started buying clothes that fit me and that suit both my body AND my personality, rather than trying to squeeze myself into things that don't work for me.

I stopped berating myself when clothes I try on don't fit. I realised that no one dress or pair of trousers can fit every person, and if something doesn't fit me, it just means we aren't meant to be paired up; just as I accept that I can't be friends with everybody, as I simply can't be right for everyone.

It has been liberating!

How can you start to accept yourself right now?

- Start small - identify some positives about yourself - your smile, your eyes, your kindness, for example. If you're stuck, as your close friends - they'll have oodles of positives about you.
- Curate your world as you want it to be - get rid of anything in your social media that makes you feel "lesser".
- Focus on your health. Not other people's. Eat the food that nourishes you, move your body in a way that you enjoy, laugh often, get outdoors, relax when you're tired. Do all those things that your body really needs from you. Treat it as you would treat a precious object. Your body is precious. It deserves all the good stuff.

- Find a colour or two that suit you so well that people HAVE TO compliment you when you wear them. A quick tip on finding these colours – sit in front of a face mirror, or on a zoom call with just yourself, and hold up fabrics of the colours you're playing with under your chin. You'll notice that some colours will drain your face of any life, and others will naturally boost your complexion. The latter are your colours. Buy clothes in those colours (hell, if you don't want to go shopping just yet, dye some old clothes that fit you but that are in colours that don't make you zing).
- Pay compliments to others. When you're in the supermarket, if you see someone in a fab skirt, tell her. If you love someone's hair, tell them. You'll start to see the power of a compliment, and the more you can give that joy to others, little by little you'll start being able to accept them back. Especially when you're wearing your colours.

And finally, remember you are perfect exactly as you are.

Notes:

What would my best friend say are my best features (either physical or personality-related)?

What do I think is my best feature?

Go through your social media and stop following any accounts that make you feel "less than".

Play around with colours. Find the ones that really make you zing.

You are perfect exactly as you are

457

CHAPTER FORTY SEVEN
Yoga - The Natural Solution for Peri/Menopause
by Julie Ann Garrido

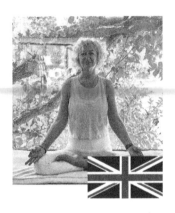

Bio: After experiencing a challenging perimenopause, Julie discovered that yoga was the natural solution that she had long been searching for. At the age of 53, she trained to become a yoga teacher, and went on to take multiple certifications including a Menopause Yoga teaching qualification. Today, she educates and teaches yoga, meditation, and wellness strategies worldwide for women in peri/menopause.

Business: Yourself Yoga & Wellness
Website: www.yourselfyoga.com

Yoga – a natural alternative to HRT? No, I didn't believe it either! But Menopause Yoga helps ease more symptoms that most other solutions, and it's all without prescription pills or supplements. Learn just how Menopause Yoga can improve your physical, mental and emotional wellbeing; enabling you to make the positive changes to your lifestyle that you never thought possible.

458

Wait, what? Yoga?? I don't think so!

Was that your reaction too when you read the title of this chapter? Because that was definitely my reaction eight years ago when I thought yoga was for anyone and everyone, BUT ME. The thought of sitting still on a yoga mat feeling all zen-like was not my cup of tea. Neither was contorting my body into unimaginable shapes and positions.

If someone had told me that it could help with my peri symptoms, my interest may have been piqued, but honestly, I would have needed some serious evidence to begin rolling out a yoga mat.

So, by now you're probably wondering how on earth did I become a yoga teacher, right? Let me enlighten you. I blame my husband (don't we all?). He was adamant that yoga would help me destress and I was equally adamant that it wouldn't. But I gave in because he promised to give it a go alongside me. The private teacher was booked to come to our home, and there was no turning back. Eeek.

Now, what happened next is difficult to describe, but I'm going with Harry Potter and his magic wand. After just 60 minutes, I felt calm, relaxed, looser, lighter, completely de-stressed, and wait for it.....HAPPIER!! I couldn't believe it. What on earth had just happened to me on that mat? My yoga journey had begun. But more than that, in many ways my life had just begun too.

Fast forward 8 years and here I am today a fully certified Menopause Yoga Teacher and Wellness Coach helping women worldwide tap into all the benefits of this wonderful ancient practice which can be a totally natural solution for peri/menopause, and an effective alternative to HRT.

Are you still with me? I hope so, for the next headline will blow your mind.

Yoga can alleviate more symptoms than most other solutions

Really?? The concept of yoga as a solution for menopause has been largely unknown...until now.

As you probably know, there are 34 official symptoms of perimenopause - the period that can last anywhere up to 10 years prior to menopause and can dog us from the age of 40, if not before.

Hot flashes, anxiety, brain fog, poor sleep, joint pain, lack of confidence, digestive disorders, overwhelm, and fatigue, are just some of not-so-fabulous delights that perimenopause brings.

However, whilst HRT may claim to be the one-stop solution for most of these symptoms, yoga can give it a run for its money too. Yoga comes in a variety of styles, and whilst all can transform our physical, mental, and emotional wellbeing, it's 'Menopause Yoga' that has the unique power to alleviate arguably many more symptoms than HRT.

How can Menopause Yoga match HRT?

Menopause Yoga is specifically designed to support women through their transition into menopause, and it combines a variety of yoga styles to address a wide array of symptoms.

Gentle flow yoga: by moving the body through a variety of poses, we can release the excess of heat that causes hot flushes, disperse the stagnant energy to lift our low moods, clear the mind to reduce brain fog, and release the knots of stress and tension to ease fatigue.

We've all seen our dogs do this pose, and for good reason. A humble *Downward Facing Dog* pictured here, has the power to

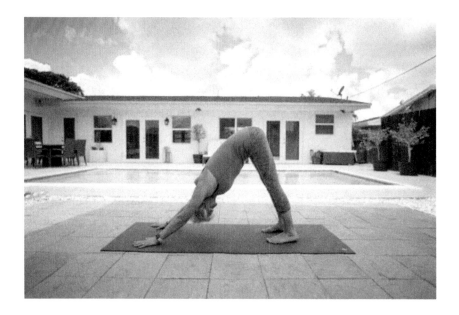

help clear our mind, alleviate brain fog, and improve memory function. But by dropping our head lower than our heart, it promotes blood flow to the brain and stimulates the pituitary gland and endocrine system – the control centre for all our pesky hormones. In addition, it gives the best stretch to the whole of the back of the body.

Yin Yoga: this passive style of yoga helps improve flexibility by lubricating our joints and fascia so that we can bend down without grunting, and maybe even reach the top shelf too. Aches and pains, joint pain, and stiffness, can all be a thing of the past with Yin Yoga.

Poses like Deer Pose pictured here, are normally held for a few minutes to enable the fascia to stretch and target deep into the hip joints. Yin also provides the ideal quiet time for rest and reflection.

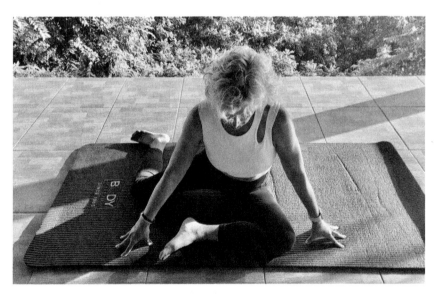

Restorative Yoga: this style of yoga is the perfect tonic for easing symptoms of fatigue, overwhelm and anxiety. By allowing the body to completely relax and surrender, it can re-energise us when menopause drains the tank. As most poses can be practised on the bed too, it makes this style of yoga one of the most popular in peri/menopause.

Poses like Legs Up Against the Wall pictured here, can provide almost instant relief to restless legs, fatigue, overwhelm, and a stressed mind. It's ideal for practicing up against the headboard too. Stay here for 10-15 minutes and feel the difference.

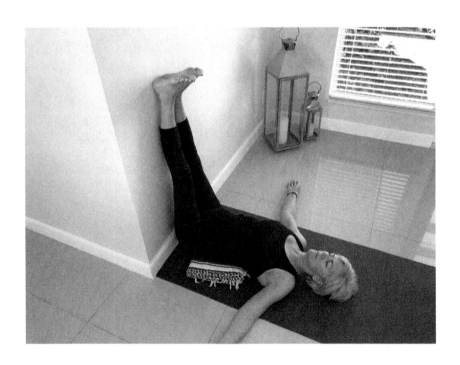

Meditation: another essential component of Menopause Yoga, meditation is a powerhouse for our mental and emotional wellbeing. By slowing down our heart rate, lowering blood pressure, and reducing the production of stress hormones, it's the perfect remedy for peri/menopausal anxiety. It's also great for alleviating brain fog and improves focus and memory too.

Meditation is not about switching off our mind, it's about simply sitting with ourselves, learning to let go, and not engaging with our thoughts. Give it a try for just 5 minutes and notice how you feel.

Yoga Nidra: known as the ultimate stress buster, and often referred to as "yogic sleep", it's claimed that ONE hour of Yoga Nidra is the equivalent of THREE hours of deep, nourishing sleep - and all without pills or potions.

By simply lying down in a cosy, comfortable position, and being guided by a specially trained voice, our brainwaves shift from their usual frantic state to a place of pure relaxation and calm, leaving us feeling less frazzled with renewed energy and self-esteem. There's only one word when it comes to Nidra, and that's WOW!

But where do I practice Menopause Yoga?

Menopause Yoga classes can be found at various yoga studios, but it's best practised online at home. That's right. You don't have to dress up and leave the comfort of your own home to enjoy this magical solution.

All that's required is a humble yoga mat, and after just 10-15 minutes of practice three times each week, you will start to see results. Yep, no one hour long classes to attend. Simply carve up your time and spread it out over the week. Your body will benefit much more by practising in this way.

How do I know this works?

Because I was so sick and tired of the lack of yoga available for women at this stage of life, I created my very own platform, *My Yoga Journey*, that is exclusively for peri/menopausal women and that follows 7 stages of guided practice and learning. Today, I work with hundreds of ladies who follow this programme at home, and the proof that it works lies in their results which are nothing short of astonishing.

"I have completed Stage 1 and I'm feeling well chuffed and have thoroughly enjoyed the last 3 weeks learning about my body. I feel stronger, fitter, and more importantly happier (I still have my grumpy days). I'm looking forward to trying a new challenge with the next stage." Rachel B.

What makes *My Yoga Journey* unique is that it's perfect for beginners and ladies of every shape and size, plus each class, tutorial, and short sequence specifically addresses peri/menopause symptoms.

Not only that, the platform comes complete with Practice

Calendars, a Progress Path, and even a Symptom Survey so that you can track the improvements in your symptoms as you progress on your yoga journey.

"My peri symptoms were mild when I started, so I was really trying to get ahead of the game on that front, but I definitely feel the benefit. I've gone from grudgingly doing yoga as it was the only exercise I could do, to it now being an enjoyable and key part of my life." Mandy M.

"My latest symptom survey has a new addition, the number 0 – seven of them in fact. This is an incredible result." Sharon M.

When would I see results?

This is the burning question, and probably the reason why HRT is so popular. No one wants to put in lots of effort without seeing results. We want to feel better NOW.

Thankfully, however, *My Yoga Journey* is a tried and tested programme that has not only brought relief to women's peri symptoms, it's changed their lives too.

Most report a dramatic improvement in their symptoms within just THREE WEEKS and by the end of the programme, many report the complete disappearance of some symptoms.

"My symptom survey is already showing 5's when they were all mainly 10's at the start and that's after just 3 weeks!! I can't wait to

see what the next stage brings." Alison T.

The ladies who have completed all 7 stages of *My Yoga Journey* have not only dramatically eased their symptoms, they've improved their mental and physical wellbeing too.

**"*I can't believe I am writing this, but I have only gone & done it! I'm so pleased to say that yoga is now a part of my life. Also, I did a check on my symptoms survey today and they have gone from mostly 3/2's to 1/0's."* Joanna B.

"Every time I roll out my mat, it leads me to conquering menopause, and my yoga practice has unlocked the door to lasting health and happiness." Beverly G.

"Yoga has taught me that I am enough, and that I can influence my symptoms with yoga. meditation, and all the tools that MYJ has taught me." Nikki C.

Yep, it seems that Harry Potter's wand is real after all!

A natural alternative to HRT

In Menopause Yoga, women now have a NATURAL solution for mastering peri/menopause that ticks as many boxes as HRT, if not more. Unlike HRT, however, it requires no medical intervention, it has no adverse reactions or side-effects, it's completely safe, and can be practised forever.

HRT is not for everyone. If there's a family history of breast cancer, ovarian or womb cancer, or even a history of blood clots or high blood pressure, HRT may not be suitable. Plus, there are women who choose not to take HRT, simply because they prefer a natural solution to help them cope with peri/menopause.

But it doesn't have to be one or the other, it can be BOTH.

Menopause is like a thumbprint and no one solution will suit everyone. However, it's high time that the ancient holistic practice of yoga is given the airtime it rightly deserves. It can be a natural and powerful alternative/complement to HRT, and a guiding light that can lead us out of a long dark tunnel.

I do hope that my story has resonated with you, and if so, perhaps you can share it with someone you know who may benefit from hearing it too?

Menopause is a natural transition at this stage of a woman's life, so a natural solution makes perfect sense. So, let me ask you this: could yoga be your natural solution for peri/menopause as it is for countless others?

Ready to take the next step? Enjoy 7 days of FREE Menopause Yoga and see what all the fuss is about. Get started with a range of 10-minute sequences to ease your worst symptoms and simply watch the magic unfold.

Dowload my free guide to starting yoga here:

Also, come join a growing Facebook community of peri/menopausal women who all practice yoga to ease their symptoms: https://bit.ly/yogaforperiandmenopause

Journal prompts:

1. Write down what's stopping you from starting yoga. Then ask yourself what's REALLY stopping you.

2. Which symptoms can yoga help you with?

3. What will be your next steps?

"To begin, begin." By William Wordsworth

CHAPTER FORTY EIGHT
Your Bedtime Routine
Begins in the Morning:
5 Daytime Strategies
for Better Sleep.
by Annika Carroll

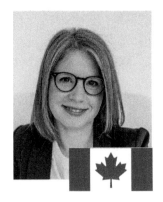

Bio: A functional health practitioner, Annika guides women to overcome sleep issues by focusing on gut health, hormones, stress, and mindset. She has battled insomnia and burnout, so she offers relatable expertise and recommendations based on functional testing and science-based evidence. She offers holistic sleep coaching options for women battling burnout, brain fog, & even… bloat.

Business: Annika Carroll Consulting
Website: www.sleeplikeaboss.com

"Let her sleep, for when she wakes, she will shake the world."
Napoleon Bonaparte

You used to fall asleep when you hit the pillow, maybe even after scrolling on your phone in bed, and you would stay asleep until just before your alarm went off.

Once we reach our 40s, finally have more time for ourselves and want to go to bed early, sleep issues appear. Sleep becomes an effort. Falling asleep and staying asleep can become challenging. When sleep isn't on point, we feel mood swings more, brain fog is substantial, and we rely on coffee and sugar to keep us going. It's frustrating because sleep is the foundation for hormone health, emotional regulation, productivity, and mental clarity.

Dr. Google tells us to have a wind-down routine, drink sleepy teas, meditate, or journal at night. And as a sleep coach, I fully support wind-down routines and calming activities in the evening.

Those are all great tips, but often not sufficient.

Why? *Because sleep hygiene isn't everything.*

Sleep during perimenopause is more complex than evening rituals like bathing or avoiding phones before bed (though they help). What we do throughout the day significantly contributes to our sleep quality. Our daytime activities impact our sleep-wake cycle, hormone release, and ability to unwind at night. This holds for all ages but is particularly important during perimenopause.

My guiding principle is: *"Your bedtime routine begins in the morning!"*

What we do during the day either adds to our sleep account

or subtracts from it. (Drinking coffee late in the day is an obvious example of subtracting from our sleep account.)

While there are lots of behaviours we engage in during the day that don't support our sleep, in addition to that, our bodies undergo systemic changes during perimenopause that can significantly affect our sleep. As our muscle mass declines, we become more metabolically unhealthy, and keeping our blood sugar stable becomes more challenging. Those pesky 3 AM wakings are often a blood sugar issue.

The decline in estrogen increases inflammation levels in the body. With that, our gut can become leaky and our body inflamed. When we have inflammation, our body releases cortisol (also at night), keeping us up. Progesterone has been declining for a while - a big player in sleep - and a hormone super sensitive to stress. Last, our liver might struggle if we're on medications, birth control, or enjoying a glass of wine regularly at night. In Chinese Medicine, the hours of the liver are between 1 AM and 3 AM.

All these changes in our bodies and the busy lives most of us lead will affect our ability to get a good night's rest.

So, how can we support a good night's sleep during the day?

Here are five things to incorporate into your routine:

1. Prioritize skylight over screen light
Is your phone waking you up in the morning, and the first

473

thing you do is reach for it to check emails or quickly scroll social media? Instead of looking at a screen light first thing, get sunlight into your eyes for 10 minutes in the morning. Sit by a wide open window or step outside for 10 minutes.

The natural light will kick in your body's cortisol production to wake you up and give you energy. And it will signal the body to set a timer and release melatonin in about 14 - 16 hours. This will reset your sleep-wake cycle, give you more energy throughout the day and help you fall asleep better at night.

It sounds too good to be true? Give it a try; it is life-changing. And what if it's cloudy? Do I still go outside? Yes, because it is 50 to 100x brighter outside than inside.

2. Timing matters with coffee

I know, I know. You need your coffee even to start thinking in the morning. But hear me out. Our bodies need time to warm up and function fully in the morning. This process is called the "cortisol awakening response". It takes about 60-120 minutes after waking for our cortisol levels to peak for the day. If we drink coffee within that time frame, our body releases too much cortisol too early in the day. Yes, that will help us get moving, but it will also lead to energy crashes earlier in the afternoon.

Often groggy when you wake up and reach for coffee or sweets around 3 or 4 PM? Get that sunlight, and the drowsiness will disappear naturally. Then have breakfast and enjoy your coffee after that. This will give you great energy for the day and enough fatigue for the night.

3. Schedule some "ME Time" for restful nights

Are you taking time for yourself during the day? Or are you giving everything to everyone but you? And then grabbing a glass of wine to unwind from the day once everyone else is in bed? No, alcohol doesn't help with sleep, but that is a story for another day.

Our bodies need to be relaxed and safe to fall asleep (this is known as the parasympathetic or "rest-and-digest" state). The best way to get there is to start putting the body into this "rest and digest' state throughout the day. We are not designed to start the day at full speed, run to lunch (on coffee), have a small break (and coffee) and then go to the evening (maybe with some more coffee or sweet snacks) without breaks.

If we do that, our brains will start processing once we go to bed and falling asleep will be difficult. We might also wake up in the middle of the night with a to-do list in our heads if we never take breaks.

But how can you build breaks into your busy schedule?

A few minutes of being in the present moment, not thinking about what to make for dinner, no scrolling on social media, no worrying. Just being in that moment. This puts your body back into a "rest-and-digest" state. And you only need a few minutes to do that. It doesn't take much time, but a conscious effort.

How can you do it?

Set a reminder on your phone to:

- Step outside for 5 minutes and take a few steps around the block
- Take 5 minutes in a toilet stall listening to your favourite song on headphones (if there is no other space to go at your work, why not go there)
- Do a few minutes of slow breathing while you wait in line to pick up your kids or waiting at the drive thru
- Have that early afternoon coffee sitting outside, and paying attention to the coffee: how does it smell? What does it taste like? How does it make me feel when I drink it?

This might sound crazy, but a few minutes here and there help your body lower cortisol levels overall and start processing what happened during the day. If we don't give our minds this opportunity, the thoughts and anxiety often come crashing in at night when we lay in bed – when it is finally quiet, and our brain begins to process.

A few short breaks during the day can help you sleep better at night.

4.   Opt for anti-inflammatory foods
Junk food can lead to junk sleep! Did you know that what you

eat during the day can impact your sleep at night? Cortisol levels need to be low in the evening to sleep well. If cortisol rises at night, falling asleep becomes difficult, and we may wake up and struggle to fall back asleep. Foods high in starchy carbohydrates (think pizza, pasta, bread, chips, donuts, bagels) spike our blood sugar.

And what goes up must come down.

To lower your blood sugar, the body releases insulin. Once insulin levels rise, the body will release cortisol to counterbalance the insulin. And if this happens too late in the evening, you won't be able to fall asleep. Cortisol is not only our stress and energy hormone but also an anti-inflammatory. When we consume a diet full of sugar and processed foods, this inflames our gut.

During perimenopause, as estrogen declines, this inflammation can lead to leaky gut syndrome, causing even more inflammation throughout our bodies. Estrogen has a protective effect on our gut that starts to lower during its decline.

If we have gut inflammation, the body will release cortisol to fight this inflammation. And as cortisol counteracts melatonin, we then have trouble sleeping. So eating a diet rich in vitamins and minerals (colourful fruits and veggies) will help keep cortisol in check and support sleep. These foods are anti-inflammatory and will prevent the body from releasing cortisol when you don't want it - in the middle of the night.

5. Skip that Peloton class

But doesn't exercise help with sleep? Yes, exercise or movement can help with sleep by making us tired. However, if you're already struggling with sleep or feeling exhausted, pushing your body with high-intensity exercise and excessive cardio can be counterproductive.

Why?

Higher-intensity exercise raises cortisol. That is why doing strenuous workouts closer to bedtime is not recommended. But if you are already struggling with sleep and energy, your body needs less of a push of cortisol from spinning on that bike or jumping on boxes. But we still need to move and maintain our muscle mass.

Doing resistance exercises or walking is excellent when sleep isn't great. Walking is highly underrated—it resets your body's inner timer through exposure to sunlight, stabilizes blood sugar, aids in fat loss, promotes cardiovascular health, and helps lower stress levels. The best part? It's free, and you can do it almost anywhere.

Incorporating these five habits into your daily routine supports a better night's sleep during perimenopause.

Give it a try for a few weeks and see your sleep and energy improve.

This way for more sleep tips....

Journal prompts:

1. One thing I did not know about sleeping better:

2. One thing I will try over the next 30 days:

3. What could get in the way of trying this? How can I deal with that?

"Life isn't about waiting for the storm to pass. It's about learning how to dance in the rain."

Glossary of terms

Hormone-related terms
- Hormone – a chemical, usually occurring naturally in your body, that makes an organ of your body do something.
- Oestrogen - Oestrogens are a group of sex hormones that promote the development and maintenance of female characteristics in the human body.
1. Estrone (E1): This is a weak form of oestrogen and the only type found in women after the menopause. Small amounts of estrone are present in most tissues of the body, mainly fat and muscle. The body can convert estrone to estradiol and estradiol to estrone.
2. Estradiol (E2): This is the strongest type of oestrogen. Estradiol is a steroid produced by the ovaries. It is thought to contribute to a range of gynecological problems, such as endometriosis, fibroids, and cancers that occur in females, particularly endometrial cancer.
3. Estriol (E3): This the weakest of the oestrogens and is a waste product made after the body uses estradiol. Pregnancy is the only time at which significant amounts of estriol are made. Estriol cannot be converted to estradiol or estrone.
- Progesterone – a hormone, $C_{21}H_{30}O_2$, that prepares the uterus for the fertilized ovum and maintains pregnancy.
- Testosterone – is a hormone made in the testes in males and in the ovaries in females.
- Grehlin – a hormone that makes you hungry.
- Leptin – A hormone made by fat cells that helps control the feeling of hunger, the amount of fat stored in the body, and body weight.
- FSH (Follicle-stimulating hormone) – a hormone produced by the anterior lobe of the pituitary gland that stimulates the growth of the ovum–containing follicles in the ovary.

- Progestins/progestogens - any of various natural or synthetic steroidal hormones, as progesterone, that cause progestational activity, used in birth control pills, in hormone therapy, etc.
- Phytoestrogen - a substance found in certain plants which can produce effects like that of the hormone oestrogen when ingested into the body.
- HRT (Hormone replacement therapy) - therapy for replacing or replenishing certain female sex hormones during menopause or after a hysterectomy.

Birth control (BC) terms
- Mirena coil – progesterone only coil, can be used as part of HRT.
- Progesterone only pill (POP) – otherwise known as mini pill.
- Combined pill – contains oestrogen and progesterone.
- Implant (Nexplanon, Implanon) – progesterone-based BC, usually implanted in the upper arm.
- Depo injection – progesterone-based BC.
- Copper coil – non-hormonal coil.

Menstrual cycle-related terms
- Menstrual cycle - the repeated process in which a woman's womb prepares for pregnancy. It ends in a period if she does not get pregnant. The menstrual cycle usually lasts about a month.
- Follicular phase - The follicular phase is the phase of the menstrual cycle, during which follicles in the ovary mature. It ends with ovulation. The main hormone controlling this stage is estradiol.
- Ovulatory phase - the second phase of the human menstrual cycle, during which the lutenising hormone surges, the follicle-stimulating hormone surges, and ovulation occurs.
- Ovulation - to produce and discharge eggs from an ovary or ovarian follicle.

- Luteal phase - the second half of the menstrual cycle after ovulation; the corpus luteum secretes progesterone which prepares the endometrium for the implantation of an embryo; if fertilization does not occur then menstrual flow begins.
- Anovulatory cycle - not involving or accompanied by ovulation.
- Amenorrhoea - a medical condition in which a woman who is not pregnant does not menstruate.

Anatomical terms
- Cervix - the narrow lower part of the womb that leads into the vagina.
- Vulva - the female external genitals.
- Vagina - the muscular tube leading from the external genitals to the cervix of the uterus in women.
- Ovaries - a female reproductive organ in which ova or eggs are produced, present in humans and other vertebrates as a pair.
- Hysterectomy - a surgical operation to remove all or part of the uterus.
- Oophorectomy - the surgical removal of an ovary.

Menopause terms
- Pre-menopause - Premenopause is when you have no symptoms of going through perimenopause or menopause. You are considered to be in your reproductive years.
- Perimenopause - the period of a woman's life shortly before the occurrence of the menopause, can last 10-12 years.
- Menopause - the time in a woman's life when menstruation ends, generally defined by having gone a year without a period.
- Post menopause - having gone through menopause.

Index

Topic	Start page of chapter(s)

Notes From The Other Side

I asked a few post menopausal women to tell me the best thing about being through this life stage. Here is what they had to say:

"Life is much better post menopause! One benefit is no cost of sanitary products. Sex can still be great!" M.L.

"Post menopause, no more periods, with the attendant tampax, pains and cramps. No worries about getting pregnant. Brain fog gradually clearing and more energy for other more interesting things" C.B.

"You can have sex whenever you want!" D.H.

"Life is so much better without the inconvenience of periods and you can wear your lovely heavy jumpers again without overheating." C.W.

"Post menopause.... everything looks the same, everything feels the same and yet, everything is utterly different. Sometimes I feel that my sexuality has just gone and that I no longer have a place/role. Other times I could kick my heels in the air (never could!) and whoop with joy that I am unshackled. Time for another adventure!" J.C.

Printed in Great Britain
by Amazon

34667961R00274